T0171537

f**P**

10 Minutes

10 Years

Your Definitive Guide to a Beautiful and Youthful Appearance

FREDRIC BRANDT, MD

FREE PRESS
New York   London   Toronto   Sydney

Note to Readers

This publication contains the opinions and ideas of its author. It is intended to provide helpful and informative material on the subjects addressed in the publication. It is sold with the understanding that the author and publisher are not engaged in rendering medical, health, or any other kind of personal professional services in the book. The reader should consult his or her medical, health, or other competent professional before adopting any of the suggestions in this book or drawing inferences from it.

The author and publisher specifically disclaim all responsibility for any liability, loss, or risk, personal or otherwise, which is incurred as a consequence, directly or indirectly, of the use and application of any of the contents of this book.

FREE PRESS
A Division of Simon & Schuster, Inc.
1230 Avenue of the Americas
New York, NY 10020

First Free Press hardcover edition April 2007

FREE PRESS and colophon are trademarks of Simon & Schuster, Inc.

For information about special discounts for bulk purchases,
please contact Simon & Schuster Special Sales:
1-800-456-6798 or business@simonandschuster.com.

Designed by Joel Avirom and Jason Snyder

Manufactured in the United States of America

10 9 8 7 6 5 4 3 2 1

Library of Congress Cataloging-in-Publication Data is available.

ISBN 978-1-439-19509-3

*I would like to dedicate this book to Dr. Harvey Blank
for teaching me to look beyond the surface of the skin;
to Sylvia Rosenthal, who is an inspiration for all things beautiful
both inside and out; to Sparky for his loyalty and love,
Maggie Maloney for directing my path every day,
and Stephane Colleu for his friendship.*

---

*I would like to thank Olivia Sanchez for her dedication, Karen Moline
for her talent and professionalism, Dominique Tinkler for her ongoing
support, and Alex Cazzaniga for his research that helped make this
book possible. I would like to acknowledge my entire Miami, New York
City, and CDI staffs for their ongoing dedication. I would also like to
acknowledge the following individuals who are important in my life:
Sam Gordon, Dr. Oscar Hevia, Alan Rosenthal, Dr. Roy Geronemus,
Misty Koons, Benjamin, Tyler, Surya, Rose Sposaro, Carl Sheusi, Kyle
White, Jan Miller, Gloria Hurtado, and the entire staff of the Four
Seasons Hotel in New York City.*

CONTENTS

PREFACE

THE RACE TO TURN BACK the clock began long before Ponce de León went off in search of the fountain of youth.

Since archaeologists began to excavate tombs of ancient civilizations, they've uncovered bones, jewelry, weapons—and beauty implements and tools, ingenious (and usually toxic) concoctions used as makeup, combs and brushes, and pots of unguents and ointments, buried alongside their owners. Tweezers, nut oils, pots of lip dyes, and recipes to combat wrinkles and pimples have been found with Egyptian mummies. Centuries later, beautifying potions were still part of a woman's daily routine, as the fabled Lola Montez revealed when she wrote *The Arts of Beauty: Secrets of a Lady's Toilet*, published in New York in 1858. Try applying a layer of beef suet to the face to help conceal wrinkles, she helpfully suggested.

Thankfully, skin care has progressed magnificently since then. When I wrote my first book, *Age-less*, in 2002, I wanted to share my knowledge about procedures and prescription products, many of which (like lasers and Botox) were brand-new and not yet well tested all over America. Since then, there's been a quantum shift not only in knowledge about cosmetic procedures, but toward a more enlightened view of what a cosmetic dermatologist can do to help you improve your appearance. Couple that with technological advances, new formulas, and new methods of delivering them, and now procedures that were once hushed up or prohibitively expensive are now discussed and accepted as part of mainstream treatments. And I think that's fantastic.

While this openness about procedures has also spawned a new generation of patients who are willing to do whatever it takes to look better, they just don't know where to start. I find that many of my patients have serious misconceptions about their skin and fear that it's too late to reverse the worst damage. (I'm happy to tell them that it's *never too late* to improve your appearance.) So even as skin care is going through an absolute revolution—and having no choice but to wash your face with plain old soap and water before choosing a greasy night cream is a thing of the past—the result is that devising a skin-care system to combat the effects of aging isn't simple anymore.

I treat dozens of patients every day in my offices in Miami and New York. Some have never seen a dermatologist before; others have already tried every possible procedure. Some patients are glowing with youth; others have already had three face-lifts before they turned fifty. Often, new patients may have cautiously tried an injectible filler, or perhaps a light or laser treatment, yet they haven't been satisfied with the results. They're thinking of doing something more intense, but they're not quite sure what.

What all these patients have in common is *confusion*.

They're suffering from a glut of too much information about aging skin. They've asked their girlfriends for advice, plied their facialists with queries, gone online and Googled countless websites and online pharmacies. They've visited the cosmetic counters, where they may have gotten conflicting advice, and scoured women's magazines, where they've read dozens of often contradictory articles, making it nearly impossible to rate or assess this information. (I believe that a little bit of quasi-accurate information is more confusing than none at all.) I can't tell you how many patients have come in with the same articles, torn out of the same magazines, yet they still don't understand the most basic, fundamental concepts about what can help them.

My patients are hardly to blame. It's next to impossible not to fall for the hype at the cosmetic counter, especially after being cajoled by skilled salespeople. "I just don't understand why I look so *old*. I feel youthful on the inside, but saggy and drooping on the outside. Can you make me look better? Not *different*," they plead. "Not like I've had anything *done*. I just want to look like myself again."

All these patients tell me that they want more than anything a simple, streamlined system to combat aging. A system that works, and works within their budgets. The reason is clear—nothing in their anti-aging arsenal has made a consistent, visible improvement in their skin's condition.

I hope you'll think of this book as the answer to all your concerns about how and why skin ages—and how best to treat it. The term I love to use to help all my patients understand skin care is "relative permanence." Even if a dermatologist injects a permanent substance to plump up your skin, it's not going to stop the aging process. There is no panacea for aging, no one product in a jar that is going to solve it all and make you young and healthy-looking again. To be blunt: No matter what you do, at the end of the day it's still all about *maintenance*. You can put a brand-new engine into a car, but eventually the brand-new engine won't be new anymore. It's going to need maintenance.

Since we're constantly aging, the secret to having great skin is both getting it *and* maintaining it, from the inside out. This book is my targeted approach to maintaining this relative permanence. You can use the information to customize your unique skin-care needs and your skin-care budget as well.

10 Minutes/10 Years is problem-driven. Part I, chapter 1 covers how skin ages, and I'll also talk about how yoga has transformed my appearance and my attitude, greatly reducing my stress while helping me lose twenty pounds and improve my skin's texture. Chapter 2 describes everything you need to know about sun damage and photo-aging. Chapter 3 tackles the newest information about sugar—and how it can age you from the inside out.

Before you decide what system you need, part II (chapter 4) provides a comprehensive guide to all the best products, treatments, and procedures that I recommend to my patients. I explain what they are and how they work—from the outside in. I list them starting with the least invasive and least expensive (nonprescription over-the-counter creams), then move on down to the most cutting-edge injectibles and laser treatments.

Once you understand the basics, you can move on to your specific area of concern in part III. You won't have to keep switching between chapters trying to figure out how to eliminate the lines around your lips or the age spots on your neck. Simply turn to the chapter dealing with whatever part of your face or body needs help, and follow my recommendations, depending on your budget and whether or not you want to see a dermatologist. Each chapter also has a list of 10-Minute Tips (most of which can be done in *much* less time), and, where applicable, 10-Minute Regimens that take less than 10 minutes to perform.

I also hope you'll refer to *10 Minutes/10 Years* as a comprehensive reference guide and basis for comparison about products and procedures prior to any visit to a cosmetic dermatologist or to the cosmetic counter. (An informed patient is always the patient best able to understand what procedures are being recommended and why.) I know that my suggestions will help you make the best decisions about how to address your unique needs.

Over the course of my career, I've changed the way I approach treating the skin. Now my approach is far more scientific. Moisturizers are far more sophisticated; their basic ingredients do more than merely hydrate the skin—they can actually help build collagen. (Think of this concept in the same vein as that of workout gear. When I was in high school, runners wore sneakers. When Adidas running shoes with a vastly improved sole became available, their speed improved and their injuries decreased. The change in materials fundamentally transformed how they exercised.) Technological breakthroughs in terms of understanding the aging process and in the manufacture of skin-care products are giving us even more tools to improve skin in the future. And, of course, incredible injectibles and other treatments can transform faces in a scant few minutes.

The happy result is that women can look far younger for their age than they did a mere decade ago. A fifty- or sixty-year-old woman today—one who looks after her skin and stays out of the sun—has skin vastly superior to that of a fifty- or sixty-year-old of twenty years before.

There's a famous Roman proverb I like: "A falling drop at last will carve a stone." It perfectly sums up the message of this book. I hope that you, too, will find the 10 minutes each day to devote to improving your skin and your life.

10 Minutes
10 Years

The Essence of the 10 Minutes/10 Years Philosophy

I CAN'T TELL YOU how many patients sit in my office and say, "Dr. Brandt, I know I'm in a rut, but I'm just too old and tired to change." That's the kind of resignation I refuse to accept—and you shouldn't either.

The truth is, these patients can't imagine how easy it is to make small, subtle changes and how quickly they'll see results if they stick to the program. They simply can't imagine that making small changes in their lifestyle and skin-care regimen will truly make a difference.

That's why I came up with the 10-Minute concept. Ten minutes isn't long. Thinking about taking a 10-minute walk isn't scary or difficult; being told to exercise an hour a day is. Start small. Set a timer. Give yourself time to adjust to change.

The key concept is *constant intervention* and *maintenance*. It's very easy to maintain a routine once you've got it figured out. Consistency counts. Sticking to a skin-care routine isn't difficult. The longer you stick to it, the easier it will become and the less time it will take (same as applying makeup or styling your hair; once you know what you're doing, it's done in a flash). Getting used to layering on different products takes only a simple change in your daily routine.

Even better—the longer you do any or all of the following steps, the easier and quicker they'll become.

The 10-Minute List

- If you devote 10 minutes a day to a quality skin-care regimen, your skin will show dramatic improvement, and you'll look years younger.

- If you devote 10 minutes a day to applying and conscientiously reapplying a broad-spectrum sunscreen, you will make a drastic difference in your skin's appearance, with less wrinkles, fewer hyperpigmentation spots, and more elasticity.

- If you devote 10 minutes a day to nutrition by reading food labels and making a conscious decision to cut down on the amount of sugar you eat, you'll feel more energetic, you'll have a better outlook on your overall health, will likely lose weight, and your skin will glow.

- If you devote 10 minutes a day to placing smaller portion sizes on your plate, you'll soon retrain your brain to know how much food you truly need.

- If you devote 10 minutes a day to yoga and conscious breathing, you will be better equipped to tackle life's constant stresses. Or you might become so enthralled by yoga that you'll devote more than 10 minutes to it— which, in the long run, will improve your energy and your sleep, giving you even *more* time to do what you love (and look great while doing it).

- If you devote 10 minutes a day to moving your body and increasing your heart rate, you'll soon discover how much better you feel, and you'll want to move your body more.

- If you devote 10 minutes a day to drinking water to which you've added a liquid green tea supplement, with potent anti-oxidant benefits, you will hydrate your body, preserve younger-looking skin, fight free-radical damage, and promote overall health.

- If you devote 10 minutes a day to doing only what you want, in peace and quiet, with no interruptions from those who need you, you'll be better able to relax, unwind, and enjoy your life.

PART I

The S Factors: Stress and Sun and Sugar

1

Skin and What You Do to It

MUCH AS WE MIGHT WISH to stop the clock, skin ages, bodies age—it's as simple as that. And considering what we do to our skin—bake it in the sun, frown, squint, pull, prod, pick, rub, blow smoke over it, or just plain old take it for granted—it remains a marvel of resiliency. Most of us certainly take for granted the miracle that is our skin, which serves vital functions, regulates body temperature, and keeps the elements out and our organs in.

Still, every woman, no matter how scrupulous she is about taking care of her skin or staying out of the sun, will start to see very subtle changes in her skin as the years go by. Sometimes slowly, sometimes with rather intimidating or alarming speed, changes become more pronounced. A typical patient in her late twenties (earlier if she smokes and/or has had excessive sun exposure) or early thirties (if she's been diligent) will become aware that, if she hasn't been paying particular attention to her skin, the bloom of youth is fading. Skin doesn't seem to be as "juicy." She may also see dryness, brown spots, an ashy tone, less resilience and elasticity, and fine wrinkles around her eyes or mouth.

"All of a sudden, I woke up and saw wrinkles all over the place," I'll hear them lament. "I need help!"

First, I joke with them that now is the time to throw away that 10X magnifying mirror—it's a lethal weapon in women's hands! Magnifying mirrors should be banished from your bathroom, since all they do is highlight your flaws so you become obsessed about the tiniest of imperfections.

Then I reassure my patients that no one ages overnight. In fact, changes in your skin occur very subtly, over time—more like a creeping progression, percolating in your skin's deepest layers. Once these changes reach a critical mass, it's akin to dumping sand on one end of a seesaw. Add a gentle trickle of sand and nothing happens; add more and the seesaw will eventually reach its tipping point. The tipping point with skin explains why you seem to notice wrinkles one day—the lines finally become deep enough to suddenly seem to "pop."

To see how you're aging, take a walk down memory lane. Pull out a picture from high school (never mind your clothes or hairstyle!) and compare it to a picture of how you look right now.

The difference between the lovely rounded cheeks you undoubtedly possessed in your high school photographs and the loss of fullness today is due to volume loss. As we age, we lose *dimensionality*. Fat deposits shift over time. This shift is an inevitable physiological phenomenon. Blame it on gravity and genetics, and realize that this explains why face-lifts don't make you look younger—only tighter. The key to restoring a youthful contour to the face is replacing this lost volume, which I'll discuss in depth in chapter 12.

Let's take a brief look at what happens to skin as you age.

Aging 101

There are two kinds of aging: *intrinsic* (biological) and *extrinsic* (environmental).

Intrinsic aging is determined by your genes, so it happens to everyone. You can't change the inevitability of this process, but you *can* slow down its progression.

Extrinsic aging, on the other hand, is entirely in your hands. Get a tan, have a smoke, stay up till the wee hours, burn the candle at both ends—and your skin is going to show it. How you expose your skin to extrinsic aging is something you have complete control over. Which is why the key to an anti-aging regimen is protecting your skin from extrinsic factors in the first place.

INTRINSIC AGING

On average, the skin covers about eighteen square feet and weighs about twenty pounds. It has two layers: the *outer epidermis*, the *dermis* in the middle, and the underlying layer of *subcutaneous fat* at the bottom. At the bottom of the epidermis, new skin cells are forming. When they're fully formed, they begin to move toward the surface. This process normally takes about two to four weeks. In the meantime, as newer cells push up, older cells near the top die and rise to the surface. This means that all the topmost layer of your skin, the *stratum corneum*, is comprised of dead skin cells.

Not surprisingly, these dead cells are still strong and sturdy enough to create the barrier layer so necessary to protect the most fragile layers underneath. But they'll soon flake off and be gone for good.

The surface of our skin sloughs off about 30,000 to 40,000 dead skin cells every minute (that translates to about nine pounds a year). But as we age, this skin-cell turnover slows down. Way down. Healthy turnover is about two to three weeks. Aging skin turnover is about two months or more. No wonder your skin looks dull and blah!

Other factors age your skin as well:

- Your skin produces fewer *collagen* and *elastin* fibers, the springy structural proteins found in bones, tendons, ligaments, blood vessels, and skin that provide natural strength and elasticity. Healthy elastin fibers can be stretched by more than 100 percent and they'll still return to their original form. Think of collagen as the basic building block that keeps your skin firm and resilient. Its destruction plays a role in the aging not only of skin, but of your entire body—which is why maintaining healthy collagen is crucial for overall health. (I'll discuss collagen and elastin in more detail starting on page 37 in chapter 3.)

- Pores are the passageways from hair follicles up to the surface of the skin. Oil-producing *sebaceous glands* are attached to pores and, much to our dismay, they grow larger with each passing year. Not only do pores get bigger, but they also become packed with dead skin cells that aren't turning over as quickly, so they look even larger.

8

- Ironically, these sebaceous glands grow larger yet produce less oil. Your skin becomes much more dry.

- The production of *melanin*, the substance that gives skin its color, also decreases.

In your twenties, the epidermis is nice and juicy, plumped up with healthy collagen and elastin in the dermis, and skin cells that easily renew themselves every twenty-eight to thirty days. Underneath the surface, however, infinitesimal changes are beginning to take place. The stratum corneum, or top layer of protective dead skin cells, thickens slightly while the skin itself starts to thin. Some fine lines may appear. Smokers and sun worshipers will notice these changes sooner, especially with lines around the eyes and lips.

In your thirties, cell turnover starts to slow down. So does collagen, elastin, and oil gland production. Skin doesn't look as fresh. It can appear blotchy, with enlarged pores and *hyperpigmentation* (brown spots). In fact, it can look downright sluggish, dull, and uneven, with more fine lines and perhaps deeper wrinkles, especially in the *naso-labial fold* (the line between the nose and the mouth). If you smile or frown broadly, you'll be able to pinpoint the areas where lines that are most likely still fairly transient will eventually deepen.

In your forties, signs of aging are inevitable. You'll continue to lose collagen and fat. Cells retain less moisture and lose their firmness, and skin can become much more dry than it's ever been. Smile or frown, and the *glabellar* (between the eyebrow) *lines* become more prominent. There are more wrinkles around your eyes and on your forehead. Hyperpigmentation spots become more plentiful as well as darker. Women in the premenopausal phase called perimenopause will start to experience subtle hormonal shifts that can wreak havoc on skin.

In your fifties, sixties, and up, the hormonal shifts of menopause, with a dwindling estrogen supply, can wreak havoc. Your skin becomes much more dry, hairs can sprout on the face, especially in the chin area (while turning white or gray on your head—charming!), and acne and the redness of rosacea can suddenly appear, particularly in the cheeks. Loss of estrogen means more skin dryness and a visible loss of luster. Skin can get rough and scaly. Fat and hyaluronic acid continue to disappear, so you can appear gaunt or sag. Jowls and under-eye bags develop, lines and wrinkles deepen and thicken, while lips thin and the chin seems more pointed. Eyelids and neck skin can look crepey and droopy too.

All this makes us look *old*. Even if we don't *feel* old.

And let's not forget gravity. It's always been there, exerting force upon our bodies; it's just that we don't have the same strength in our skin and bone structure to withstand it effectively as we grow older. This is especially true for those women whose skin tends to sag, so their features (foreheads, eyebrows, under-eye bags, jowls) appear to move on down, much to their consternation.

To add insult to injury, once we stop growing, our skeleton that supports our skin starts shrinking. Calcium supplements help, but that's not the whole answer. The size of your face eventually shrinks (called *bony reabsorption*) over time as well. Earlobes seem to grow, not just from the weight of earrings over the years, but also from lost volume and resiliency. Noses also start shifting down. And, think about it—if you lose volume in your face, making it smaller, your nose *is* going to look bigger; it's like painting a picture on a smaller canvas. So you're not going crazy if you think your nose is turning into Pinocchio's—everything is relative!

But take heart, as there are plenty of things you can do to stave off your biological destiny—and turn back the clock.

EXTRINSIC AGING

While scientists and physicians haven't figured out how to stop intrinsic aging, extrinsic aging is another story altogether. This is both good and bad. Good if you've used sunscreen religiously and taken care to stay out of the sun, have never smoked, watched your weight, exercised regularly, eaten a healthy diet, minimized stress whenever possible, and gotten enough sleep. Bad if you haven't!

Extrinsic aging is a result of your own habits: sun exposure, an unwholesome diet (especially an overconsumption of sugar, which I'll discuss in chapter 2), lack of exercise, not getting enough sleep, and stress. Equally important is your attitude toward aging and how you manage your daily life. The old chestnut "You're as young as you feel" is really true. If you *feel* old, how can you *look* young? And if you're going through a bad patch in your life, the pressure you're under is going to show, too.

10

Even small changes in bad, even entrenched, habits can reap large rewards in your skin's appearance.

Sun Exposure

The worst (and yet most easily correctable) of these bad habits is allowing your skin to be exposed to the damaging ultraviolet radiation of the sun, day in and day out. An astonishing four out of five wrinkles are directly caused by sun damage alone. I like to kid my patients that the only day they don't need to wear sunscreen is during a hurricane—but, in truth, there's not much to laugh about when it comes to sun damage.

Not surprisingly, there is often a disconnect between a woman's biological age and her skin's appearance when these women have spent many years in the sun. I've seen patients in their late forties or early fifties who come in, shaded by broad sun hats and swathed in scarves, and look decades younger than many of my smoking, sun-worshiping patients in their late twenties and early thirties. Take a good look at the skin on your buttocks, which has had next to no sun exposure throughout most of your life, and you can see what skin protected from the sun looks like—smooth, unwrinkled, and unmottled by hyperpigmentation. So smokers and tanning bed junkies are almost always chronologically older than their biological age.

I've found that few of my patients truly understand (or want to believe) just how accelerated their aging is due to sun exposure, or how to find the right sunscreen and use it properly. I always tell them that, frankly, there's no point in spending thousands of dollars on advanced treatments if they're going to immediately undo what they've just paid for—by going right back out in the sun without adequate protection.

The absolute easiest and least expensive way to prevent photo-aging is to use a good, broad-spectrum sunscreen every day and apply it properly. It takes only a minute or so. Not only will it save you thousands of dollars in skin-care products and treatments over the years, but it may well save your life. Skin protected from the sun is much less likely to develop skin cancer.

I'll discuss sun damage, called photo-aging, in depth in chapter 2.

Fredric Brandt, MD

Sleep Deprivation

Sleep deprivation is reaching epidemic levels in America, and nearly a quarter of all American adults use some sort of narcotic sleep aid, such as Ambien, to help them fall asleep. Few get the necessary seven to eight hours of deep, uninterrupted sleep that bodies need.

During sleep, our bodies secrete growth hormones and replenish cells and tissues. Skin that's mercifully not assaulted by the daytime barrage of free radicals has time to replenish itself. Cortisol, the hormone that helps regulate body maintenance (and stress management), is secreted early in the morning. Studies have shown that if you go to sleep before midnight, you secrete more growth hormone during the wee hours. Go to bed at three in the morning and get up at noon . . . well, it's not the same thing. Over time, this can accelerate the aging process throughout the body. If, on the other hand, you stick to a regular sleep schedule and get the amount of rest your body needs, it will affect your hormones in a positive way.

Without enough sleep, you are tired, irritable, sluggish, and more prone to depression and stress, leading to a weakened immune system—and it shows. Don't forget that the skin is the body's largest organ, and as the largest source of elimination (through sweat) it reflects what's going on inside. Just take a look in a college dorm during finals, when students are pulling all-nighters to study. Even young adults, who normally have faces free of wrinkles, will look like hell when they don't get enough sleep, with waxy, blotchy complexions, breakout clusters, and deep, dark circles under their eyes.

Bottom line: Make your bedroom a haven from the stress of daily life and get some sleep. When you do, you're improving your skin with the absolute least amount of energy possible! Adequate, refreshing sleep is without question the easiest thing you can do to stimulate the production of growth hormone, help your body function better, and help your skin look better, too.

Smoking

Here's my recipe for instant aging: Go to a tanning salon with a cigarette.

If that doesn't work, bake your skin to a crisp on a beach with a cigarette!

My patients who are smokers are usually astonished when I ask them how long they've been lighting up as soon as they sit down in the examining room. Even when they lie (as they often do, since they're ashamed they're unable to quit), I can always tell a smoker's face, as certain markers are visible to my trained eye.

The toxic chemicals in cigarettes (acetone, ammonia, arsenic, benzene, lead, mercury, and tar) and cigarette smoke (gases such as carbon monoxide, formaldehyde, hydrogen cyanide, and nitric oxide) interfere with the microcirculation of blood and nutrients to the skin. There's a sharp drop in collagen production, causing a loss of firmness. Nicotine constricts small blood vessels, so less oxygen is available to nourish the skin.

As a result, smokers have a particular yellowish-ashy tint to their skin that makes them look hard and older. Their skin is dull and sallow. They get more blackheads; their collagen decreases and their pores become enlarged. The dirtiness of smoke lands right on their faces (whether they think it does or not). They have crow's-feet around their eyes, from squinting. And they have fine lines around their lips from all the pursing activity, so the area around their mouths and noses usually looks pretty awful. In fact, a Korean study reported in the *International Journal of Dermatology* in January 2002 reported that current smokers have a higher degree of facial wrinkling than nonsmokers and past smokers. Fortunately, heavy smokers who finally stopped smoking had fewer wrinkles than current smokers, but microscopic, or as yet unseen, superficial wrinkling was evidenced in smokers age twenty to thirty-nine.

Nicotine also blocks estradiol, a form of estrogen in the skin. (This may also explain why smokers often have a harder time getting pregnant.) With less estradiol, skin becomes drier and thinner. This may explain why women tend to have smoker's face more visibly and sooner than men who've smoked for the same amount of time.

Smoking also wreaks havoc on the internal organs, especially the lungs. Smokers' cells can't regenerate as quickly. They bruise more easily, bleed more during surgery, and take much longer to heal. This can have dire consequences for anyone contemplating surgical procedures to improve their appearance.

I tell my patients that I know that nicotine is exceptionally addictive—more so, even, than opiates like heroin, or crystal meth, or alcohol. Few of my patients want to keep smoking; they confide that they've tried everything—acupuncture, nicotine patches and gum, hypnosis, you name it. It's hard for any dermatologist to see anyone suffering from an addiction, especially when the patient knows full well what damage is being caused.

The best way to deal with smoking is to treat it as you do sun exposure: Don't start in the first place. If you smoke now, try your utmost to quit. Smokers who manage to stay off cigarettes notice improvements in their skin almost immediately.

Stress and How to Manage It

No skin-care system will work on the outside unless you're willing to work on the inside as well.

Stressing over your age is a surefire way to look and feel old. And if you *feel* old, you will *become* old. I've certainly treated enough unhappy patients to see firsthand the havoc wreaked upon their skin by emotional turmoil. When stressed, your body releases *cortisol,* a hormone that causes a spike in your insulin level, which then triggers mood swings and sugar cravings. Many who confide in me during their appointments try to spin a layer of positive thinking on what's going on in their lives, but with just a few gentle questions I can see what's lurking underneath: mountains of negative thinking. Confronting and uprooting those mountains take work, effort, and often involve some emotional pain. But in the long run it will be worth it—not only for your skin, but for every aspect of your well-being.

There are two aspects to this kind of work that have helped me tremendously, and I have no doubts that they can help you too.

I'm living proof of how a body-mind system can have transformative results. I'm always working on myself. I need to do this work, not only to keep myself healthy, but also to keep up my energy when dealing with the dozens of patients I treat every day. What keeps me going is that I truly love my work. I love meeting new patients and seeing old ones. I love educating them about the best skin care, and I love helping them look their best. I love doing the research about new products and technology. I love developing a skin-care line with wonderful properties and ingredients.

Loving your work and finding contentment in your life are profound aspects of healthy, vital living, but they're often overlooked and underrated. Happiness manifests itself in your appearance—just take a look at wedding photos or new parents cooing over their babies. It's not a cliché to say that skin glows when people are happy, no matter what their age.

But even those who thrive in a high-pressure profession, as I do, have to manage stress. Sure, stress is a part of life, and some days are better than others, but my patients don't come to me to be confronted with my worries. If I'm tense, it shows in the clenched muscles of my face. That anxiety will immediately transfer to my patients, making them anxious, too, and harder to treat (especially with needles!).

So I made a conscious decision years ago to figure out how to manage my stress—not on a temporary basis, but on an ongoing, daily basis that demanded commitment. I explored all the options in terms of exercise, diet, and holistic treatments, and decided upon a basic, sugar- and gluten-free diet (which I'll discuss in chapter 3), yoga (which I'll discuss in the next section), meditation, and acupuncture.

Commitment is something you can't buy. It's a crucial component to both managing stress and improving your skin. Countless patients have come into my office wanting a quick fix for all their skin concerns. Yes, I can often give them nearly instantaneous improvements with a wide range of injectibles, but it's up to them to take the time to *commit* to sticking to my recommended maintenance program.

This is especially true with OTC (over-the-counter) skin-care products. Anyone starting a specific skin-care regimen should see some results in a month. (After all, you can't undo a lifetime of skin abuse overnight.) But only by sticking to a new regimen religiously and as directed for *at least twelve weeks* will you begin to see *profound* results.

The Wonder of Yoga

I used to enjoy pounding my joints while jogging on the streets, and many of my friends swear by running and other forms of intense aerobic exercise. What works best for me, my body, and most especially my skin is yoga.

Even with my jam-packed schedule, I make time for yoga five to six days a week, for at least one to two hours every morning. Clearing my day to slot in my yoga practice is not a luxury; this is a crucial aspect of maintaining my health.

There are so many aspects to yoga and its benefits that most novices don't know about, especially now that yoga is considered trendy and something that celebrities boast about—even though it's been around for a mere five thousand years! Yoga in its purest form not only opens up channels of energy in the body and realigns the joints and organs, but with what's called *Pranayama*, it trains and liberates the breath. It improves concentration, clearing all extraneous junk from the mind when you enter a meditative state (this is called *Samadhi*). I've found yoga to be fantastically calming, and when I enter the Samadhi state, it helps me manage my stress in ways I never could have before. And at the same time, it is also remarkably energizing, giving me what's akin to a turbo-charged effect. It's as if I'm using the "exhaust" of having done the yoga postures and breathing to fuel and propel the *next* experience. Anyone who does yoga on a regular basis will undoubtedly experience these states as well.

My yoga teacher and trainer, Carl Sheusi, sees his clients literally transformed by a commitment to yoga. "Often, they'll come to me and say, 'Okay, well, I mean, you know, I want to do this posture, I want to learn this style of yoga, I want to lose weight, and get more flexible. I'm looking to do all these things,'" he told me. "My response is, great! You'll get that. But you're going to get so much more because you've come to the wish-fulfilling tree. And that tree is the source of all things—which is within you. My job is simply to give it back to you. What you're looking for isn't out there, it's already *inside*."

Yoga wakes up the subtle energies in the body, energies that have stagnated from either misuse, lack of use, or some form of trauma (such as tight connective tissue and muscles). The proper form and the positions in yoga allow those energies to flow unimpeded, bringing about a vibrant state of relaxation and well-being. And since your circulation will improve, it naturally follows that your skin's appearance will, too.

Remember that your skin is the largest organ of elimination in your body. Yoga helps to eliminate toxins, through sweat and through the exhalation of breath. Once you become better at it, it will also bring an incredible suppleness and elasticity to the joints, the internal organs, and certainly to the skin.

Aside from the physical benefits, yoga helps me think. The meditative aspect to my yoga practice helps me focus and brings me awareness. This becomes an amazing tool in my life, allowing me the opportunity to make changes that I hadn't been aware of before (because I didn't know I could experience them).

I believe that this wonderfully calming meditative aspect to yoga—the bringing together of body and emotion into a profound sense of *mindfulness*—is as important as what you eat or what treatments you use on your skin. While meditation is a wonderful tool when you're stressed, it's something that you can apply all day long. If something happens in your office or your home and you feel yourself about to flip, try to take a step back. Focus your thoughts, use calming breathing techniques, and your stress will become more manageable.

Of course, I don't want to imply that your skin won't look wonderful if you don't want to incorporate yoga into your life. I grew up with parents who ran a candy store, and trust me on this—I never thought I'd become a yoga devotee in my forties. I didn't realize just how much I needed yoga until I began to devote more time to it. (And finding the time to commit to this kind of mind-body exercise was the first step in making my body as healthy as it could be.) For me, it's a profoundly important weapon in my anti-aging arsenal.

It takes a very healthy mind-set to commit to a yoga practice. As with everything that involves serious work and challenges, changes will not happen overnight, but they *will* happen. Systematically, over a period of time, we can literally transform our minds and bodies. When the body is less toxic, the mind becomes less toxic, and then everything else in your life can change, too.

Carl recommends that beginners to yoga start with whatever level and frequency makes them feel comfortable. (Needless to say, you need to discuss any exercise program with your physician prior to starting.) There are many different kinds of yoga—Ashtanga, Bikram, Integral, Iyengar, Jivamukti, Kripalu, Sivananda, and Viniyoga, to name a few—with different emphases. Some are more attuned to the spiritual/meditative aspects, and others are more physically challenging. Some move at a slow, contemplative pace, and others are aerobic and intense workouts.

When you first begin your yoga practice, challenge yourself slightly, but don't overdo it, as you might injure yourself. Injuries can happen to those who are inexperienced yet who can't help comparing themselves to more flexible, experienced classmates. Don't judge yourself against anyone else if you take classes. Set your own goals and work at your own pace.

And enjoy it!

10-Minute Tips

- Make a list of all your habits that contribute to extrinsic aging: smoking, stress, sun worship, not getting enough sleep, et cetera. (This should only take a minute—hopefully, less!)

- Then take 10 minutes to figure out how to undo each habit. Write this down. Keep it in the back of your mind. Even if you can spend only 10 minutes a day undoing a habit, that's enough of a start to keep you going.

- Go to bed 10 minutes earlier each night until you're getting enough sleep.

- Buy several bottles of sunscreen at a time and keep them in the house, office, and handbags. Reapply often.

- Spend 10 minutes taking a break from your family or other demands and sit somewhere quiet where you can relax in peace. Set a timer so everyone knows that this 10 minutes belongs to you—and don't give in before the 10 minutes are up!

- Stay away from secondhand smoke.

- Stretching for a few minutes every morning or even mid-afternoon will give you an energy boost.

- Do 10 minutes of yoga to start. If you can't get to a class, watch a video. Start slow.

2

(Don't) Let the Sunshine In

THERE'S A FAMOUS SONG at the end of the now famous musical *Hair*, commonly referred to as "Let the Sunshine In." Of course, actually letting the sunshine in—onto your skin—is anathema to dermatologists. So it's rather ironic that the real title of this song is "The Flesh Failures (Let the Sunshine In)"— which pretty much sums up how I feel about what happens to your skin when you get a tan!

Sun exposure gives you wrinkles. Sun exposure makes you look old. Furthermore, there's no such thing as a healthy tan. A tan is a response to injury; it's the way our body protects itself from sun damage. Which is why tans are not proof of glowing health, but visible evidence of DNA damaged on a cellular level as well as shredded collagen and elastin.

That sun exposure can also kill you when melanoma rears its ugly head seems almost beside the point. Right?

Of all the things you place in your anti-aging arsenal, protecting yourself from the sun is the easiest, the cheapest, and the quickest weapon you'll always have. It works. It has no side effects. It's proven.

So why are so many of my patients who do know, deep down, that the sun fries their skin, baking on the beach? (Especially in Miami, where sun exposure is a year-round problem.) I always tell them that, frankly, there's no point in spending thousands of dollars on advanced treatments if they're going to immediately undo what they've just paid for—by going right back out in the sun.

Do they listen? Some of them do. Sadly, some of them don't.

Photo-aging is the term used to describe how the aging process is accelerated by exposure to the sun—and you don't get this exposure only when you're relaxing by the pool. It happens when you walk from your car to the mall, or out shopping, or when driving, or when taking a healthy walk. Plus, photo-aging is exacerbated by the dire fact that there is less of the protective ozone layer in the atmosphere than there was a few decades ago, so the sun is more potent.

The result? Fine lines, wrinkles, dryness, roughness, precancerous lesions, and larger pores. Photo-aging also affects elasticity, so your skin will become looser, less pliable, and more likely to droop. Photo-aging is also directly responsible for "sun spots/age spots," or freckles, those large brown spots and dots (properly called *hyperpigmentation*) or white spots and dots (*hypopigmentation*).

What's so obviously apparent is that sun exposure causes skin damage to appear decades earlier than it normally would. One reason is damage caused by *free radicals.* Free radicals are molecules with an unpaired electron, made naturally as a by-product of oxygen consumption. Since it has just one of the two electrons it needs, the molecule becomes unstable while it seeks out its mate. In the process, it attacks other molecules in an attempt to snitch one of their electrons. The result is damage to collagen and elastin.

And, as you'll see in the next chapter, a phenomenon called *glycation,* which prematurely ages the skin, is caused by eating sugar and intensified by sun exposure.

For a visible reminder of this phenomenon, take a look at the French actress Brigitte Bardot in her heady days of youth, with creamy, unlined, glowing skin. Now take a leap forward. Several decades later, her face is still beautiful yet ravaged by photo-aging. And she can hardly be faulted for this. When she was young, no one knew how pervasive and progressive sun damage could be.

My patients come face-to-face (literally!) with the amount of photo-aging they've undergone when they sit down in front of a machine I have in my office. Developed by Procter & Gamble, who developed the database and license the analysis software, the VISIA Complexion Analysis System is a computer that takes high-resolution digital photographs of your skin and prints out photographs of your skin spots, pore size, texture, wrinkles, evenness, trapped bacteria, and UV damage. After comparing them to thousands of others with your same age, gender, and skin type in the database, it gives you an instant ranking of how progressive (or not) your overall facial skin damage is.

Many of my patients, especially those in Miami, are positively shocked when they see the extent of the damage. I've found that once they finally realize what they've done to their skin, they're finally ready to stop sunbathing or ducking into the tanning salon for their weekly touch-up. Or perhaps they've spent a lot of time and effort on top-quality OTC products, or doctor visits for expensive and invasive treatments, to no avail. Their skin is dull, dry, blotchy, and riddled with hyperpigmentation spots, and they come to me for an assessment of their regimen. I tell them that nothing will really work if they undo its effects by immediately going back in the sun.

Other patients are more nonchalant, shrugging and telling me something along the lines of "Oh well, I guess I've been a bad girl and abused my skin, so it's too late to do anything about it." I hasten to tell them it's not true. It's never too late to change your habits!

I've always believed that tanning has an addictive quality, because so many of my Miami patients claim to do their best to stay out of the sun, but just can't manage it. Their problem is more pervasive than merely keeping up with American society's misguided cultural bias that tans make you look thinner or healthier—almost as if they're "tanorectics." (Never mind that in most Asian countries, women do their utmost to stay out of the sun, prizing a pale skin tone above all others, the cultural bias of which is beyond the scope of this book.) Tanorectics are never dark enough. They can't see that their skin is fried to a crisp, or how the wrinkles become more etched with every passing day. They can't seem to stop.

My gut feeling has now been substantiated, with a study recently published by researchers at Wake Forest University Baptist Medical Center. They were surprised when their study showed that the UV rays in tanning beds appeared to trigger the production of *endorphins*, the chemicals in the brain linked to pain relief and euphoria, such as "runner's high."

"We had previously shown that ultraviolet light has an effect on mood that tanners value," the head of the study, Mandeep Kaur, MD, said. "Now, in this small study, we've shown that some tanners actually experience withdrawal symptoms when the 'feel-good' chemicals are blocked." Some tanorectics literally do suffer from nausea, jitters, anxiety, and other cold-turkey-type symptoms when they suddenly stop tanning. These symptoms are akin to what drug addicts feel during withdrawal. It would also explain why tanorectics don't stop tanning even though they've been told countless times that they're greatly increasing their risk of developing skin cancer and they're absolutely increasing their risk of looking prematurely aged.

Fortunately, determination and a willingness to rethink this addiction can change a tanorectic into a person who shuns the sun—and looks and feels much better as a result. What's needed is a new sun lifestyle, one that's not about the sun at all but about avoiding it whenever possible. And one that includes hats, scarves, sunglasses, umbrellas, SPF clothing, tinted windows in your car, and a commitment to using them.

Even though I spend most of my time in Miami, I'm living proof that you can live in a hot climate without tanning, burning, blistering, and wrinkling!

Let's take a look at what sun can do to your skin.

FITZPATRICK SKIN TYPES

Dr. Thomas Fitzpatrick developed this classification system based on the amount of pigment in skin in order to calculate the skin's burn rate. Knowing a patient's skin type helps dermatologists choose the best procedures to treat sun damage.

Types I and II are most likely to have suffered or will suffer severe sun damage. Those with more natural pigment in their skin, such as Types V and VI, tend to age better as their skin has an innate SPF of 6 to 8. Everyone on this list, however, needs to protect their skin from UV radiation.

TYPE I   Extremely fair skin. Always burns, never tans.

TYPE II   Fair skin. Usually burns, tans minimally.

TYPE III   Medium skin. Sometimes burns, often tans gradually.

TYPE IV   Olive skin. Rarely burns, tans easily.

TYPE V   Dark skin. Very rarely burns, tans profusely.

TYPE VI   Black or dark brown skin. Never burns, tans very easily.

About Solar Radiation

The sun is a great big ball of gas flinging toxic ultraviolet (UV) radiation out into space. UV rays are classified by wavelengths (nanometers, or nm) into three types: UVA (400–320 nm), UVB (320–290 nm), and UVC (290–200 nm, which is absorbed in the atmosphere). The shorter the wavelength and the lower the number, the greater the energy level of the light. Most of the UV rays that bombard us are UVA, with a small amount of UVB.

No one, no matter what your skin tone, is immune to damage from UV radiation.

First, there is *oxidative stress*, where DNA and tissue damage occur along with cell death and even skin cancer.

Second, heat and *thermal stress* cause loss of proteins, which is responsible for cell protection against external stressors.

And third, there is *hydric stress*, where the skin is unable to retain water, causing dehydration.

When damaged, skin increases the production of a pigment called *melanin* to protect skin cells from damage. (This is the same pigment that already colors your hair, eyes, and skin.) Extra melanin darkens the skin so it becomes tanned.

Getting a tan offers next to no protection from further UV damage, as the extra melanin provides no more than a Sun Protection Factor (SPF) of about 2 to 4. The minimum recommended SPF is 15—and this only refers to burning UVB rays, not aging UVA rays.

UVA is the aging ray. Although it doesn't cause burns, the UVA ray's longer wavelength makes it far more intense than UVB's, and it allows these rays to penetrate deeply into the dermis, down where our DNA lies. (This is where the cancer risk comes into play.) There, it ravages collagen and elastin and stimulates production of the pigment-producing *melanocytes* responsible for hyperpigmentation spots, wrinkles, and uneven skin tone.

There's no escaping UVA. It's present every day whether or not you're baking on the beach. It can penetrate glass, so it's as essential to protect yourself while driving or while working in sunny rooms as it is when you're trekking across the desert. Tans may fade, but the aftereffects of UVA exposure can last forever.

UVB is the burning ray. It's most potent between 10 a.m. and 4 p.m., which is why I always tell my patients to avoid or minimize exposure during these hours. UVB cannot pass through glass and has a more superficial penetration into the skin—but it's still enough to trigger free-radical damage. The result is lines and wrinkles, as well as a propensity to develop precancerous lesions and skin cancers.

It's equally important to protect your eyes from the sun. Too much UV radiation can damage the cornea and lead to cataracts, a clouding of the lens of the eye that can cause blindness. Not all tinted glasses, even those that are very dark, have a protective effect, as UV filtration is the result of an invisible chemical applied to the outer surface of the lenses. Check the label or ask your optometrist about your options.

Sunscreen Is a Must

If you apply only one product to stave off the years, let it be sunscreen.

Anyone who cares about preventing wrinkles and maintaining an even skin tone must wear a sunscreen with an SPF (sun protection factor) of at least 30 every day, no matter where they live or their daily routine. The SPF rating is calculated by comparing the amount of time needed to produce a sunburn on protected skin to the amount of time needed to cause a sunburn on unprotected skin. For example, let's use a fair-skinned woman who would normally turn red after 10 minutes in the sun. Ten minutes is her "initial burning time." If she uses a sunscreen with SPF 2, it takes 20 minutes in the sun for that person's skin to turn red. Now, if that person uses a sunscreen with SPF 15, it multiplies the initial burning time by 15, so it will take 150 minutes, or two and a half hours, for that person's skin to turn red.

Sun damage doesn't occur just from lying on the beach while vacationing in the Caribbean. It happens all the time: winter and summer, sunshine and rain. Even fluorescent lightbulbs emit UVA rays that break down collagen and elastin.

I always wear sunscreen, even if I'm just popping out for a minute to run an errand, and I prescribe the same for all my patients. Remember that sun exposure doesn't come only from above; snow, sand, water, and even concrete

Fredric Brandt, MD

reflect UV rays, and clouds don't block them, so you can get sunburned on a cloudy day.

Sunscreen blocks UV rays from penetrating the skin. But the biggest misconception is that a regular sunscreen with a high SPF will effectively protect you from both UVA and UVB. In truth, in America, SPF only measures protection against UVB, meaning you can gauge how long it may take to get sunburned. The FDA does not require a quantitatively equivalent measure of UVA, the aging and cancer-promoting ray. The system in Europe is different, and UVA protection is measured with an *IPD*, or immediate pigment darkening, number. The higher the number, the better the protection. There is also a scale to measure UVA protection in Asia, called the PA scale, with three different categories: PA+, the level of UVA protection from 0 to 4; PA++, the level from 4 to 8; and PA+++, the level greater than 8. That the FDA has not mandated a UVA-rating system like that here in America strikes me as an egregious dereliction of duty.

Most sunscreens use two types of active ingredients: chemical blockers, to absorb ultraviolet light, and physical blockers, to reflect ultraviolet light back into the environment. Do bear in mind that no sunscreen can completely protect you from harmful UV rays, but it can drastically reduce their effects if used properly. Check the sunscreen label for broad-spectrum ingredients, which should provide protection against UVA and UVB.

UVA chemical blockers are anthranilate, avobenzone (Parsol 1789), and benzophenone. Recently approved by the FDA is Mexoryl, an effective UVA blocker used in most other countries and soon available in America.

Physical blockers of UVA and a small amount of UVB include zinc oxide and titanium dioxide.

UVB chemical blockers are the cinnamates (octylmethyl cinnamate and cinoxate), octinoxate, oxybenzone, Padimate A, Padimate O, and sulisobenzone. PABA, once commonly used, is no longer available because it caused allergic skin reactions.

Many of my patients have complained over the years that sunscreens are chalky, or that they heat up the skin, or that they caused shine, clogged pores, and breakouts, especially in those with oily skin. That has been true, especially as chemical blockers absorbed the sun's heat, which could lead to redness and discomfort. But the micronization process has improved consistency by breaking up the goopy zinc oxide or titanium dioxide particles that left streaks and clogged pores, and using better chemical blockers such as Mexoryl can take the heat away.

These ingredients do work, but clients still want something better. As I said, no matter what sunscreen you use, you're never going to get 100 percent protection from UV radiation. For the UVA and UVB rays that do reach the skin, you need to have some form of protection and repair from the free-radical damage that occurs at a cellular level.

Most consumers don't understand what sunscreen is and how to use it. They think it's only meant to be used when you're "going in the sun"—at the beach or while on vacation, for instance. But everyone needs to get the message that sunscreen is as much *a daily* necessity as brushing your teeth and washing your face and hands.

So I thought about how "sunscreen" is really a misnomer, and instead recommend products with additional ingredients that offer daily UV protection. They not only filter and block UVA and UVB radiation, but they also trigger the skin's defense mechanisms. By doing so, these "sunscreens" are as much treatments for the skin as they are protection from damage *before* it occurs.

Ingredients you should look for include: avobenzone (Parsol 1789), octinoxate, octisalate, and oxybenzone for UVA and UVB protection; Imudilin, which restores and stimulates immune defense mechanism; Alistin, an antioxidant with a repairing effect that prevents cell death and loss of proteins; GPS, a moisturizer that protects cells from losing water; DSBC, a free-radical scavenger that also acts as an anti-inflammatory with soothing properties; and a combination of green tea, white tea, and grapeseed extract, powerful antioxidants that fight free-radical damage with anti-inflammatory properties.

For the most effective use of any sunscreen:

- Always apply sunscreen at least 20 to 30 minutes *before* going outside. The active ingredients need that time to become *active*.

- Always apply at least one teaspoon of sunscreen to the face. Don't forget your ears, nose, and neck. One of the most common problems with sunscreen use is how little is put on. Measure out a teaspoon until you're able to eyeball it, or use an amount equivalent to the length of your index finger.

- If you're going to the beach, or playing an outdoor sport, you need about one ounce of sunscreen to cover yourself adequately. Most sunscreen bottles come in either an eight-ounce or twelve-ounce (the size of a can of soda) size, so you'd be using either one-eighth or one-twelfth at a time.

- Sunscreen *must* be reapplied every two to three hours when you're outside. It degrades in sunshine and heat and *stops* working. So if you're planning to spend the day outside, you should go through at least half a bottle of sunscreen if you're using it properly. The less sunscreen you're wearing, the lower the SPF. This helps explain why so many people who do use sunscreen at the beach can't understand why they still end up freckled and fried.

- Some sunscreens are labeled as being water-resistant. These sunscreens stay on the skin longer even if they get wet from pool water, ocean water, or sweat. But water-resistant doesn't mean *waterproof*. Water-resistant sunscreens still need to be reapplied after you go swimming, for instance, so check the label for reapplication times. The effectiveness of a sunscreen is reduced if it's applied incorrectly or if it's washed off, rubbed off, or sweated off.

- Sunscreens degrade in heat, so stashing bottles of them in a car that will bake in a parking lot all day will make them quickly lose their effectiveness. Keep sunscreen in a cool environment—preferably not the bathroom!

- Be sure that your sunscreen is broad-spectrum, meaning it has both UVA and UVB protection. The only way to trust that it truly is broad-spectrum is to read the label carefully. By law, active ingredients such as chemical blockers must be listed at the top of the ingredient list and labeled as such, along with their percentage. I recommend sunscreens that contain avobenzone (Parsol 1789) and/or zinc oxide or titanium dioxide for UVA and some slight UVB protection, as well as at least one chemical UVB blocker, such as a cinnamate or oxybenzone.

- You need at least an SPF of 30, whether you're playing golf or walking to the store. Doubling the dose of a product with an SPF of 15 will *not* give you the protection of a 30! It's heartening to see some of the largest cosmetic companies coming out with new sunscreens that have SPFs of 40 and higher.

- If you have sensitive skin, you may have to resort to a sunscreen without chemical blockers, since they may be irritating. Try those with zinc oxide and/or titanium dioxide.

- Many makeup products claim to have an SPF of 15 or 20. This is a great idea in theory, but SPF can refer only to UVB blockers. In addition, moisturizers and foundations are absorbed by the skin, so they are by nature less effective than sunscreens at sitting on the skin's surface. No cosmetic should ever be used in place of a good broad-spectrum sunscreen.

- One of the excuses I often hear from those who skip the sunscreen is that they're working on their vitamin D production. While sunlight does help in vitamin D's synthesis in the body, all you need is about 10 to 15 minutes of unprotected sun exposure over a very small area of your body for this to happen. Anyone who eats a healthy diet and takes a good vitamin supplement has no need of sun-created vitamin D. If you're not convinced, don't forget that the sun hits every part of your body, so wear sunscreen on your face, neck, and arms, and expose your legs or feet to the sun for 10 minutes. That will be more than sufficient!

- Sunscreen is an absolute must after any dermatologist treatments, such as lasers and microdermabrasion, that sensitize your skin. You can actually become severely burned if you don't completely shield your face. Be sure to ask your dermatologist if you need to take extra precautions. If you take prescription retinoids, you also must use sunscreen, as the sun can intensify their side effects, leading to intense dryness, redness, and flaking.

- In addition, certain medications, such as antibiotics, also increase sun sensitivity, leading to potential rashes, irritation, or severe sunburns. Ask your prescribing physician or pharmacist and follow their directions. And don't forget to read the labels of any OTC drugs or products you might be using, and note if there are any warnings about sun sensitivity. If you notice any symptoms after being out in the sun, contact your physician and/or pharmacist immediately for advice. Make it a rule to buy a new bottle of sunscreen every time you pick up your prescription!

ABOUT SKIN CANCER

There's no excuse for the terrifying rise in the amount of skin cancers in this country. As you age, about 65 percent of melanomas and 90 percent of basal and squamous cell skin cancers can be attributed to sun exposure.

There are three main types of skin cancer: melanoma, basal cell carcinoma, and squamous cell carcinoma. They're typified by moles or freckles that change shape, color, texture, or get crusty and bleed. Basal cell and squamous cell carcinomas are usually called non-melanoma skin cancer.

Basal cell cancer is the most common and easiest to cure. It usually appears as small, fleshy bumps or nodules. It's followed by squamous cell cancer, which usually appears as nodules or as red, scaly patches that can spread into different parts of the body. Melanoma, the least common but the most lethal cancer, spreads down into the body, making it the most difficult to excise and cure. An early-stage melanoma often appears as a tiny light brown to black flat mark. A fourth type of growth, *actinic*, or *solar*, *keratosis*—usually called precancerous lesion—is also something to monitor closely. These lesions are usually scaly, pink, or sandpapery spots, which sometimes form a crust on top. The crust can peel off and then re-form. There are more than 5 million diagnoses of actinic keratosis each year in America.

According to the American Cancer Society, most of the more than 1 million cases of non-melanoma skin cancer diagnosed each year are considered to be sun-related. Melanoma, the most serious type of skin cancer, is being diagnosed more frequently than any other cancer. It will account for about 62,190 cases of skin cancer in 2006 and most (about 7,910) of the 10,710 deaths due to skin cancer each year. According to the Centers for Disease Control and Prevention (CDC), the death rate from melanoma in the United States has been going up about 4 percent a year since 1973.

Even more shocking is the fact that skin cancer is the most common type of cancer in our country—one in five Americans will develop skin cancer in their lifetime—yet the easiest to prevent. According to a report in the April

2006 issue of *The Mayo Clinic Health Letter*, your risk of the disease doubles if you've had five or more sunburns over the course of your lifetime. Like tans, sunburns, called *erythemas*, are proof of short-term sun damage and a response by the skin to overexposure to UV radiation. Each tan and each burn increases the risk of skin cancer. The damage is cumulative—just like wrinkles, hyperpigmentation, creases, and blotches are cumulative, too.

Just as many long-term smokers never develop lung cancer, many long-term sun worshipers never develop skin cancer. The specific trigger or predisposition hasn't been discovered yet, which is even more reason to use a good sunscreen blocking both UVA (aging/cancer promoting) and UVB (burning) rays—and to stay out of the sun as much as possible, particularly during the peak hours of 10 a.m. and 4 p.m. Never leave the house without sunglasses with a UVA/UVB rating of 99 percent or higher, an opaque hat with a large, wide brim so the back of your neck isn't exposed, and an extra bottle of sunscreen. (Straw hats, which are quite porous, aren't as effective as hats made from tightly woven or thicker fabrics. And baseball hats only shade part of your face, leaving your neck and ears completely exposed.) If you love outdoor activities, such as swimming or golf, you can find clothing made from tightly woven fabric, called Solumbra, with special fibers that give it a built-in SPF that endures through hundreds of washings and days in the sun, as well as rinses such as Rit Sun-Guard, added to the laundry that can make any fabric more sun-resistant.

You may also want to try Heliocare supplements. Heliocare is a daily oral supplement made from an extract of the plant *Polypodium leucotomos* (PL), a type of fern. Researchers at Harvard realized that it works as an anti-oxidant that decreases the photo-toxicity of UV radiation. Although not FDA-approved, Heliocare has been used in Europe for twenty-five years and is presumed safe. It is not a sunscreen and should be taken as an adjunct to daily sunscreen use. Remember that you should always discuss whether or not supplements are right for you with your dermatologist and/or physician.

Make a habit of seeing a dermatologist at least once a year—and more often if you spend inordinate amounts of time in the sun—for a complete body check. Any suspect spot, or one that's changed shape or itches or bleeds, should be examined as soon as possible. If cancer is suspected, a simple biopsy is required. When detected in its earliest stages, skin cancer is often curable. When melanoma spreads, it often is not.

Fredric Brandt, MD

About Self-Tanners and Other Sunless Tanning Products

Sunless tanners, sometimes referred to as self-tanners or tanning extenders, have been promoted as a risk-free alternative to baking in the sun. They contain an FDA-approved color additive called dihydroxyacetone (DHA) that reacts with amino acids in the dead skin cells (the stratum corneum) on your skin's surface to stain it. The stain will "take" according to how well and how evenly exfoliated your skin is and to how evenly the product is applied. (There's a large potential for streaking and stained palms, so follow directions.) The effect is temporary, lasting anywhere from a few days to a week. They contain no SPF, so they're not a replacement for sunscreen.

They may sound good in theory, but I don't recommend self-tanners, because they reinforce the myth that tan = healthy.

Even though DHA has been approved for topical use, there are restrictions. According to the FDA, DHA should not be inhaled, ingested, or used in such a way that the eyes and eye area are exposed to it because the risks, if any, are unknown. This can be risky as many of my patients and countless others like to visit salons and spas for spray-on applications of DHA. Some of them have told me that they've had brown-stained urine after a session with the spray. This is extremely alarming, as it means that DHA has been absorbed into the bloodstream.

If you do get spray-on tans, be sure to ask the salon or spa if your eyes and eye area will be protected; if your ears, nose, and mouth will be protected; and if there is any possibility of inhaling the DHA solution. Your eyes and all mucous membranes must be covered completely. Breathe through your nose during the treatment.

If your questions are not adequately answered prior to treatment, run out the door and find a salon or spa that will take better precautions.

Another (alleged) tanning substance that is banned by the FDA is canthaxanthin, the ingredient found in imported "tanning pills." Although the FDA has approved canthaxanthin for use as a color additive in food, if used sparingly, it should never be ingested in the larger amounts found in OTC supplements. Side effects can include liver damage; a severe itching condition called *urticaria* (hives); and an eye disorder called *canthaxanthin retinopathy*, in which yellow deposits form in the retinas.

Other lotions and pills claim to be "tanning accelerators" that work by stimulating and increasing melanin formation in the skin. They usually contain the amino acid tyrosine, along with other substances. According to the FDA, these products are ineffective and unapproved drugs. As such, they should not be sold.

THE KILLER TANNING BED

Tanning salons like to trumpet the "fact" that they're safe because only UVA radiation is released. How wrong they are!

According to the FDA, tanning beds and lights are just as dangerous as tanning at the pool or on the beach. Not surprisingly, the UVA rays emitted by a tanning lamp or bed are often far more intense than those produced by the sun. The aging and cancer risks associated with outdoor tanning are the same as tanning in a salon. For these reasons, neither the FDA nor I will recommend the use of indoor tanning equipment — ever.

Worse, researchers at the Mayo Clinic, as reported in April 2006, found that the percentage of women under the age of forty with basal cell cancers tripled between 1976 and 2003, while the rate of squamous cell cancers increased fourfold. An unusual finding was that only 60 percent of the cancers appeared on the head and neck — the most obvious place, as these parts of the body are the most exposed to the sun. The other 40 percent appeared on the torso.

The likely culprit? Tanning beds. The likely reason? Tanning beds most often use UVA. "Occasional yet intense UVA exposure poses a greater risk of melanoma skin cancer than does spending long hours in the sun," claimed the researchers.

If for whatever deluded reason you do decide that you must visit the tanning salon, be aware that the FDA has a radiation safety performance standard for sun lamps, so there must be a warning label, an accurate timer, an emergency stop control, an exposure schedule, and protective goggles. *Always* wear the goggles, use short exposure time, and stick to the time limit for your skin type. And then ask yourself why you're ruining your skin and quite possibly your life in the misguided notion that a tan makes you look better.

Fredric Brandt, MD

10-Minute Tips

- Cancel your appointment at the tanning salon.

- Convince all your tanorectic friends to cancel their appointments at the tanning salon.

- Put gloves on while driving. (Keep them stashed in the car.) "Driving gloves" with little holes in the leather look attractive, but are not ideal for protecting all the skin on your hands.

- Reapply sunscreen to hands after you wash them. Keep a bottle near the sink.

- Read active ingredient labels on each bottle of a new brand of sunscreen you're considering.

- Make sure it provides *both* UVA and UVB protection.

- A teaspoon of sunscreen is all you need for your face.

- Get in the habit of applying sunscreen half an hour before you leave the house or office.

- Buy a hat with a wide brim, made from thick, opaque fabric, that completely shields your face and neck.

- Do an online search for attractive and practical clothing made from Solumbra.

- Change all the halogen lightbulbs in the house and replace with standard bulbs.

- Change your schedule to ensure you spend the least amount of time outside during the peak sun hours of 10 a.m. to 4 p.m.

- Tint the windows of your car, if possible.

- Protect yourself from the sunlight that comes through the windows of your office.

3

Sugar: The Enemy Within

SUGAR DOESN'T JUST MAKE you fat.

It doesn't just do terrible things to your internal organs. It doesn't just pre-dispose you to type 2 diabetes and a host of other ills.

Sugar also ages you. From the outside in as well as from the inside out.

According to the latest statistics compiled by the Centers for Disease Control and Prevention (CDC), an astonishing 60 million American adults are obese; the percentage of adults considered obese has doubled since 1980. There are 9 million children considered to be overweight, which puts them at risk for developing health-related issues as they grow older. It is projected that around 4.7 percent of our population will be diagnosed with diabetes by 2010. These figures are shocking. Worse, officials are claiming that the current young generation might actually have a shorter life span than their calorie-shunning, bicycle-riding, video-game- and Big Mac–deprived grandparents.

Still, if anything good is to come as a result of the raging obesity and dia-betes epidemics in this country, it might very well be the broadening research into the role of sugar and its effects on the aging process—its addictive proper-ties, how it's metabolized, what it does to the body, and how it affects your skin.

As I mentioned in the last chapter, my parents ran a candy store when I was growing up in Newark, New Jersey. When I was little, there was nothing I loved more than stuffing myself with sweets. Candy made the day complete.

I managed to keep my sweet tooth in check as I slimmed down as an adolescent, knowing that I had to take better care of myself. But I wasn't prepared for the *huge* improvement I saw in my skin as soon as I went on a fairly restrictive diet in 2002, the hallmark of which is no refined sugar. Not only that, but I gradually lost twenty pounds, have more energy than ever, and have managed to keep these pounds off. Patients who haven't seen me for a while all ask if I've had a "little work" done to my face, because my complexion is so much more vibrant. And I tell them, yes, I have. I've "done" a new eating regimen that's sugar-free. It's a lot cheaper than a face-lift, with much longer lasting results!

First, let's take a look at how eating sugar can affect your skin, and then I'll discuss my recommendations for removing sugar from your diet, as well as my advice on what supplements can help improve your skin's appearance (and which are a waste of money).

The Glycation Phenomenon

Some of the most fascinating research currently under way targets a phenomenon called *glycation*. This research seeks to explain the physiological principles behind the damage to the circulatory system caused by inflammation in diabetics. Aside from causing a host of severe medical problems and complications, severe cases of diabetes—particularly type 2, caused by excess weight and sugar consumption—can necessitate toe and foot amputation as well as lead to blindness and premature death. Researchers wanted to know why these specific kinds of changes were happening in the body, and where all this micro-inflammation originated. Once they got down into the molecular level, they saw what was happening: the aftereffects of the glycation process.

There are two types of glycation: *endogenous* (inside the body) and *exogenous* (outside the body).

ENDOGENOUS GLYCATION

In the body, endogenous glycation is a natural process where sugar molecules in the blood and in the cells chemically bond to protein fibers and to DNA, changing their shape and properties. The sugar literally sticks to the proteins, in the

Fredric Brandt, MD

process eventually forming harmful new molecules called *advanced glycation end products*, or AGEs for short. (Ironic acronym, isn't it?) These AGEs accumulate, causing inflammation and damage to nearly all the cells and molecules in the body. As a result, they're extremely important and worrisome factors in the aging process.

Since collagen is the most prevalent protein in the body, approximately 70 percent to 75 percent of the skin's dry weight, it is subject to AGE damage. Elastin, the protein fiber in the dermis that also provides elasticity to the skin, is also prone to AGE damage. Once damaged, by an irreversible process called *cross-linking*, the naturally springy and resilient collagen and elastin become stiff and brittle.

The last thing you want your collagen to become is brittle. Then it cracks. For instance, think about what happens when you smile—if you have normal, healthy collagen and elastin. As your smile fades, your skin snaps back to its original position. If your elastin is brittle and prone to snapping, your skin can't snap back. The collagen isn't plumped up enough to support it. Skin will sag. It will look *old*.

Glycation also affects what type of collagen you have. There are several kinds of collagen, the most abundant being Type I, Type II, and Type III. Type III is the most stable and longest-lasting. Glycation reduces Type III collagen into Type I, which is more fragile and less stable than Type II or Type III. When that happens, your skin looks and feels less supple, and is more prone to wrinkling.

Your glycated collagen is the unseen enemy within. I like to think of it as akin to a toxic landfill that causes wrinkles, sagging, a loss of resilience, that haggard look on the outside, and the development and exacerbation of many chronic age-related diseases on the inside.

EXOGENOUS GLYCATION

Exogenous glycation was first described by French scientist Louis Camille Maillard in 1912. He discovered how the amino acids in proteins bind to sugars during cooking and baking. The resulting reaction caused the food to turn golden brown. AGEs formed when any food with sugar was combined with proteins or fats and cooked over heat. The higher the temperatures and the longer the cooking, the more AGEs would form. Any foods that are browned, such as baked goods (especially if they've been caramelized), commercial french fries (to which sugar is added to make the fries look better), beer or colas (with their appetizing caramel hue), or barbecued meat (cooked over intensely hot fires) will be high in AGEs.

Conventional wisdom used to disregard exogenous glycation. Scientists thought these food-based AGEs were not absorbed during digestion and were simply excreted. But it turns out that this is dangerously wishful thinking. In fact, the AGEs you eat in the form of sugar not only will make you fat or predispose you to diabetes, but they may also play a major role in the development of debilitating and fatal diseases (and, of course, play a major role in the aging of your skin). That cake you have baking in the oven may have a gorgeous golden brown crust, but inside each delicious crumb is a time bomb in the form of these AGEs.

Bottom line: A diet high in sugar, especially in foods with the sugar-protein-heat combination, can cause premature aging. Or worse.

When I first started reading the research, I was skeptical. As I studied it in depth, however, I became shocked. The facts about glycation and the damage caused by AGEs were incontrovertible. Of course, I knew that any excess consumption of sugar wasn't good for your health, but I hardly thought that excess consumption of sugar-laden foods high in AGEs could have a detrimental effect on skin.

For that reason, glycation isn't just a buzzword, or a fad overhyped by skin-care manufacturers. It's science, backed up with research by those trying to save the lives of the millions of Americans diagnosed with diabetes and age-related illness each year.

The good news is that you can take a proactive approach to the glycation issue. When it comes to your skin, you can marvel at the wonders of technology and use topical products that target these AGEs and work from the outside in. You can restrict the amount of sugar you eat and be more mindful of how you cook and what kinds of AGE-heavy, processed foods you'll buy (see "AGEs in Food").

AGEs IN FOOD

A diet devoid of sugary processed foods and low in fat will automatically reduce the amount of AGEs you're ingesting. A study headed by Teresia Goldberg, RN, a research dietician, for the American Dietetic Association came to the conclusion that "diet can be a significant environmental source of AGEs, which may constitute a chronic risk factor for cardiovascular and kidney damage."

The foods with a combination of fat and protein (such as baked goods) show the highest AGE levels. Roasted nuts are high in AGEs; raw nuts less so. In addition, the method of cooking is also a risk factor. Although red meat doesn't contain sugars, barbecued red meat has the highest AGE levels, followed by broiled or roasted; boiled or stewed over low heat has the lowest. Highly processed food is also suspect. A slice of toast has a low level (30 kU AGE/serving), while a similarly sized portion of toasted rice cereal has 600 kU/serving. It's thought that the processing of prepared food, at very high temperatures, inflates the AGE levels. So does their extrusion process, by which foods are reduced to small pieces in production.

To lower your risk of AGE consumption, reduce consumption of these foods:

- Full-fat cheese
- Butter
- Red meat
- Highly processed foods, especially cereal, baked goods, and snack foods

Change your cooking methods. Try to stew, poach, boil, or cook over low heat for longer periods. When possible, avoid high-heat methods such as:

- Barbecuing
- Broiling
- Searing

- Roasting in a very hot oven

- Caramelizing

  Instead, eat a diet rich in:

- Low-fat dairy

- Fish

- Fruit

- Vegetables

- Whole grains

Tackling AGEs with Skin Care

The more I read about glycation, the more determined I became to create products that would help my patients (and everyone else) minimize its effects in the body and on the skin. And I know I'm not alone. Several other cosmetics companies, including Estée Lauder, Avon, and Guinot, have created their own lines as well. As I'll show in the sections on OTC collagen and anti-aging creams starting on page 58 in chapter 4, there are effective, FDA-approved products that have been proven to create new collagen.

But what's the sense in building new collagen if it will quickly become brittle and stiff? If you can find a way to destroy the AGEs, on the other hand, the new collagen will be healthy and supple. This is where the technological development of new substances as well as the improved synthesis of old ones put those in the know on the forefront of skin care, creating new over-the-counter creams with ingredients unheard of only a few years ago. One of these ingredients is called Alistin, an anti-oxidant with anti-glycation properties, as well as a repairing effect that prevents cell death and collagen loss.

What will have the most potent effect is a synergistically designed collagen-building regimen:

Fredric Brandt, MD

- First, you *repair* the old, brittle Type I collagen, which breaks down into harmless amino acids and is excreted.

- At the same time, you *prevent* more damage by *protecting* your skin from the sun's harmful radiation with an effective sunscreen.

- Then you *replace* it with supple new Type III collagen.

- Next, you *remove* excess sugar and other AGE-laden foods from your diet.

- Last, you *strengthen* your new, improved collagen—and keep it strong.

In other words, you'll be improving your skin from the outside (with a skin-care regimen) as well as from the inside (by cutting down on sugar).

Equally important is the strengthening of your elastin fibers. Elastin is often overlooked and ignored in skin-care products, but without strong and resilient elastin fibers, you won't have a desirable, firm tone to your skin. It can't snap back easily. (People born, in rare cases, without elastin have skin that can only hang slack.) So you'll get more value from your skin-care regimen when you repair and strengthen both your collagen and elastin.

Weaning Yourself Off Sugar

How myriad the delights of sugar! Sweet, delicious, soothing—it was probably the first therapist on our planet, easing our worries as we bit into another delicious morsel.

I grew up surrounded by sugar. We didn't eat fast food, but what a special treat it was for me and my brother to accompany our mother to the deli, where we gorged ourselves on pastrami sandwiches and french fries twice a month. And we had cake for dessert every night. My father was a diabetic who didn't take care of himself or modify his diet as well as he could have, and he died way too young from renal failure.

Even knowing I have a genetic predisposition to diabetes didn't stop me from indulging my sugar cravings. Let me tell you, it hasn't been easy to wean myself off my addiction. Because I *was* addicted. Not to expensive Belgian chocolate or to piping-hot cinnamon buns (you know, the kind you smell in the airport that automatically make your mouth water, even if you've just eaten a seven-course gourmet dinner). I was addicted to Orangina soda and to chocolate soy ice cream. The more sugar you eat, the more you need. And so the more I scarfed down my frozen delight (a whole container at a time, I'm ashamed to admit) and the more soda I drank, the more I craved them. As a result, the endless sugar cycle continued.

It was only by going cold turkey on my sugar cravings that I was finally able to realize just how much better I felt and looked without junk sugar in my life. As soon as the sugar went in the garbage, the garbage went out of my system. I stopped putting excess AGEs into my body. I lost twenty pounds. And I looked completely rejuvenated.

On top of the physical cravings for sugar, there's the other issue of using food as solace and that depriving yourself of comforting food is tantamount to depriving yourself of emotional succor. After all, how many of us grew up having our parents reward us with dessert ("Eat all your vegetables and you can have a cookie!") or a treat ("Be a good girl and you can have a candy bar!").

I believe the concept of deprivation is the reason most diets fail, since dieters (subliminally or overtly) think of food deprivation in the same manner as emotional deprivation. *Diet* is a failure word. As soon as you get on one, you want to get off. In addition, the word *diet* implies a temporary situation, one that you're changing in a negative way. Restricting what you eat may be positive for your body, but it's still a negative emotional way of eating; by their very nature, diets make you think about what you *can't* have. What I'd like you to do is strive to change your emotional reward system. And realize that a healthy diet free of extra sugar is more rewarding—not just physically, but emotionally too.

Another thing you can do is take a good hard look at your habits. What do my patients say to me?

Committing yourself to healthy eating habits is like committing yourself to yoga or another exercise program. Making a conscious, concerted effort to remove excess sugar from your life is all about change: changing an unhealthy habit—one that ages you—and changing your emotional patterns. When you do this, you're jumping outside the box, shifting from a physical diet to an emotional well-being diet.

Fredric Brandt, MD

SUGAR LURKING EVERYWHERE

Surprisingly, many prepared foods contain hefty amounts of sugar. Learn to read labels and see how many grams of sugar are in each serving. Food manufacturers often cleverly try to hide the fact that sugars are in their products, so don't be deceived if you don't see "sugar" or "sucrose" on the label. The following list shows just how many types of sugar there are:

Barley malt, blackstrap molasses, brown sugar, cane sugar, corn syrup, date sugar, dextrose, fructose, fruit sugars, glucose, glucose polymers, high fructose corn syrup, honey, invert sugar, lactose, maltitol, maltodextrin, maltose, malt sugar, mannitol, maple sugar, raw cane sugar, sorbitol, stevia, and turbinado sugar.

What you're saying is, I need to have wellness and a healthy approach to eating be a part of my daily life. Of course, I hope you'll start using an anti-glycation skin-care regimen, but putting on a cream is a lot easier than modifying your diet. For optimal results, you'll want to prevent new damage, repair old damage, strengthen new collagen and elastin, and keep as much excess sugar and AGEs as possible out of your body.

ABOUT SUGAR AND CARBOHYDRATES

Many people don't understand the basics of nutrition, or of weight loss, and it's certainly not their fault. Seemingly every month some new diet comes out, or the principles behind some old diet are contradicted.

The simple truth is this: If you eat more calories than you expend, you *will* gain weight. And if you eat foods with minimal nutrition, laden with fat and sugar, and spend little time burning calories through exercise, you not only will gain weight but you will gain it with alarming rapidity.

The American obesity epidemic is extremely scary. Small children who are already overweight, and whose bad eating habits are reinforced or ignored by their parents, are likely to grow up to be obese adults with a host of infirmities and a shorter life span. It is amazing when you think that the average family is absolutely vigilant about what kind of premium fuel to put in their cars, whereas the fuel they put into their bodies—the food they eat and the beverages they drink—is junk, devoid of nutrition and laden with garbage calories.

Nearly every food is some form of a carbohydrate, and carbohydrates have sugar in them. This isn't necessarily a bad thing, as your body metabolizes carbohydrates to provide the energy that keeps you alive.

Carbohydrates are found in the following food categories: dairy, fruit, legumes (beans, lentils, soy, et cetera), nuts and seeds, starches (grains, flour, potatoes, corn), sugars (table sugar, honey, fruit sugar, or fructose, et cetera), and vegetables.

Whenever you eat, your pancreas releases a hormone called insulin to regulate your blood sugar levels. The *glycemic index* measures how your blood sugar level changes whenever you eat different carbohydrates. Food with the highest glycemic index (sugars and starches) cause the highest release of insulin. When your insulin level rises, your blood sugar level *lowers*. This explains how the cycle of mindless eating can endlessly repeat itself: When you eat foods with a high carbohydrate level, your blood sugar goes up. You feel great. Your belly is full. Then insulin is pumped out and your blood sugar goes way down. Wham. You get hungry. You may feel jumpy and anxious. You have to eat. So you eat more carbohydrates—anything to fill the hunger.

Eventually, those who continually overeat, especially sugars and starches, tend to have an enormous glycemic load over time, leading them to become insulin resistant, which in turn can lead to type 2 diabetes, where insulin is no longer produced in sufficient quantities, or not used efficiently.

Type 2 diabetes is nearly always caused by lifestyle—poor diet and lack of exercise contributing to obesity. Everyone should worry about diabetes, even if you think you have no risk factors. Due to the obesity epidemic in America, type 2 diabetes is currently growing at an annual rate of about 9 percent. At this rate, there will be more than 100 million people with diabetes and another 100 million with prediabetes in the next twenty-five years. Taking care of these diabetics' medical needs will become an impossible task for an already overburdened health care system. And no price tag can be put on the misery they may suffer when their health deteriorates.

Type 2 diabetes is so dangerous because too much glucose in the bloodstream wreaks havoc wherever it goes. The circulatory system, eyes, kidneys, and blood vessels can become damaged, leading to heart disease and hardened arteries, retinal disease and glaucoma, kidney failure, and other problems. Circulation is compromised, leading to nerve damage in the feet; some are severe enough to warrant amputation.

The reason I state this so bluntly is simple: What are the primary components of blood vessels, through which our blood passes?

Collagen and *elastin.*

So if excess sugar and AGEs damage the collagen and elastin in your skin, they will damage the collagen and elastin in your blood vessels, too. Unlike skin damage, however, it is nearly impossible to repair collagen and elastin damage to blood vessels once they've become compromised.

According to the Centers for Disease Control and Prevention (CDC):

People with type 2 diabetes have high rates of cholesterol and triglyceride abnormalities, obesity, and high blood pressure, all of which are major contributors to higher rates of cardiovascular disease. Many people with diabetes have several of these conditions at the same time. This combination of problems is often called *metabolic syndrome* (formerly known as Syndrome X). The metabolic syndrome is often defined as the presence of any three of the following conditions: 1) excess weight around the waist; 2) high levels of triglycerides; 3) low levels of HDL, or "good," cholesterol; 4) high blood pressure; and 5) high fasting blood glucose levels. If you have one or more of these conditions, you are at an increased risk for having one or more of the others. The more conditions that you have, the greater the risk to your health.

In addition, high blood sugar causes your body to lose fluid. Less fluid means less hydration, which means drier skin. Dry skin is often itchy and irritated and cracked. Scratch it and it can start to bleed. Open wounds can get infected. And diabetics with high blood sugar take longer to heal because the excess sugar feeds the bacteria causing these infections. As a result, the infections are not only worse than normal but take longer to heal.

10-Minute Tip

Where skin is concerned, higher levels of insulin cause inflammation and can prematurely age skin. Diets low in sugars, starches, and processed foods, and high in fresh fruit, vegetables, whole grains, and low-fat protein can regulate your blood sugar, keeping you on an even keel, full of energy, and at far lower risk for developing type 2 diabetes, heart disease, high blood pressure, circulatory diseases, and many other conditions.

As soon as you cut down on sugar, you'll see an improvement in your skin. Instead of rewarding yourself with a candy bar, think about rewarding yourself with new, improved skin and a longer, healthier life.

THE BRANDT CLEANSE

My friends and colleagues who've followed my progress as I weaned myself from sugar thought at first that I was being too restrictive, even starving myself. But I eat a *lot*. The difference now is that I eat *healthy*. And, frankly, you can only eat so much when you're eating healthy because you've utterly lost your cravings for sugar and junk food.

This is the cleanse I started, devised by my chef, and my acupuncturist, Reula Kameron. Reula told me that I needed to follow this for only a month, and I made a commitment to stick to it, because it was for a short time. The first few days were horrible, and I was sorely tempted to cheat, but I stuck it out. Actually, I was very skeptical when I first started the cleanse but was astonished when I felt not just slightly better, but transformed. At the end of the month I felt so much better, with so much more energy and a clearheadedness I hadn't felt in a long time, that I simply could not go back to my old way of eating and my Orangina fix. I refused to add processed sugar back into my diet so I could become addicted again.

Now, years later, I'm still on the cleanse, and it's become my daily diet. Despite once being so addicted to sugar, I find it remarkably easy to stick to. I occasionally relax some of the rules and eat different fruits or some cheese. Once in awhile I'll even have dessert. But you know what? Anytime I now eat sugar, it's unbearably, cloyingly sweet. I never thought I would so completely lose my taste for it—but I have.

This cleanse basically works to rid your body of the *Candida albicans* yeast bacteria that thrives in our intestines. Candida feeds on—you guessed it—sugar. In a healthy gut, there is a proper balance of the candida and the acidophilus bacteria, which plays a necessary role in digestion. But because the average American eats a diet laden with sugar, the candida flourishes and overwhelms the delicate bacterial balance necessary for optimal health. Worse, candida can invade the rest of our bodies, eventually landing in the brain. A candida overrun is one reason why those who eat a lot of sugar usually feel slow and sluggish. Sometimes there is memory loss or forgetfulness. A cleanse will jump-start your sugar-free life.

Before beginning any diet, especially a cleanse, be sure to inform your physician. Anyone with preexisting medical conditions, or who is pregnant or breast-feeding, should never start any kind of diet without medical supervision.

NOT PERMITTED

Wheat in any form

Any grains with gluten

Yeast

Refined sugar in any form (table sugar, honey, maple syrup)

Juice

Dairy

No root vegetables (such as potatoes or beets)

Most fruit

PERMITTED

Fish, shellfish, meat

Non-roasted nuts and seeds

Gluten-free grains (such as millet and spelt)

Vegetables (except root vegetables such as potatoes and beets)

Green apples

Blueberries

Be careful when doing the cleanse that you don't end up eating sugar in a different form. If you've removed all fruit except apples and blueberries, don't let yourself eat five apples or a quart of blueberries a day. Or lots of yeast-free bread. That's a signal your tenacious candida is making a last-ditch effort to survive. Try not to give in. Eat something savory, like a handful of cashews, when you feel a sugar craving coming on. See recipes beginning on page 233 for a seven-day meal plan for the Dr. Brandt Cleanse Diet.

Boosters for Health: Supplements

When I was studying to become a physician, I worked as a cancer researcher at Memorial Sloan-Kettering Hospital, where I studied the properties and effects of natural anti-oxidants and how they could fight the damage to skin caused by free radicals. Free radicals are a highly reactive oxygen species, imbalanced molecules that are the naturally occurring by-products of a normal metabolism process called oxidation. Because free radicals steal electrons from healthy cells to neutralize their own charge, they'll attack cells and prevent them from functioning properly, interfering with DNA and collagen synthesis—which translates into premature aging. Free radicals have also been implicated in degenerative diseases and cancers.

In addition to your body's own production of free radicals, they're also created by our environment, which causes reactions in the skin. Free radicals can be generated during sun exposure as well as by cigarette smoke, environmental pollutants (such as smog), chemicals, and other toxins.

The way to combat free-radical damage is with anti-oxidants. They have the ability to prevent the free radicals' chemical reactions from occurring in and harming the skin. The way they work on the skin is to interfere with these chemical reactions, thereby stopping them from taking place. And there's another technology, with the use of tiny spheres called *fullerenes*, which literally absorb the free radicals in the skin. Instead of merely blocking the chemical reaction, they actually scavenge them up and collect them.

Since I've always been particularly interested in how natural anti-oxidants function, as well as how chemically synthesized ones work, of course, I concentrated my research on green tea, white tea, and grapeseed extract. These three ingredients are chockful of anti-oxidants. They're good for your body, and they work from the outside in. But that isn't enough. There are also many supplements that will help you fight free-radical damage from the inside out. This is why I devised liquid supplements to help fight free-radical damage from the inside out as well. Unlike pills, which contain binders and fillers that can interfere with their absorption and potency, a liquid supplement is directly absorbed by your body.

Fredric Brandt, MD

VITAMIN AND MINERAL SUPPLEMENTS
FOR OPTIMAL SKIN

Although anyone who's seen my vitamin bottles at home knows that I've always been a big fan of good supplementation, I'm always amazed when my patients dump a bag of their supplements during an appointment and explain that they've gotten their advice about which vitamins to take from a helpful salesclerk in a health food store. Of course, some salesclerks are extremely knowledgeable about nutritional supplements and proper dosages. But many of them are not.

Seeing a competent nutritionist to discuss your diet and what your body needs is always a good idea, especially as we age. Our bodies' nutritional needs change over time, so it's much smarter to get qualified advice during an appointment or two than waste your money on supplements you might not even need or be able to metabolize properly.

I recommend the following vitamin and mineral supplements for optimal skin vitality. Take one each day. Be sure to ingest only the best-quality supplements, as the vitamin industry is not regulated by the FDA, and cheaper brands often contain less of the ingredients than claimed on the package. Read the labels carefully to ensure you're taking the recommended dosage. Some vitamins (such as vitamin A) can be toxic over time if ingested in large quantities, so pay attention to the FDA recommendations and do not self-diagnose. I always insist that my patients see a qualified nutritionist to discuss supplements. The dosage can vary tremendously among individuals, so each regimen should be different. Dosage may also be tailored to other health issues as well as how much you weigh. In addition, if you're taking any prescription medications, supplements may potentially interact with them, so always mention any supplementation to your physicians, just to be on the safe side.

For overall health	1 multivitamin/mineral pill	
For improvement of hair and nails	Biotin	2.5 to 5 milligrams
For cholesterol	Omega oils	1000 micrograms

For cell growth and heart health	Coenzyme Q	1000 micrograms
For anti-oxidant protection	Vitamin A	1,000+IU
	Vitamin C	1 to 3 grams
	Vitamin E	1000+IU
For help with healing and improving the skin's topmost layers	Zinc	10 to 30 micrograms

10-Minute Tips

- Use anti-glycation or other collagen-building and strengthening treatment creams every day.

- Use sunscreen and avoid sun exposure.

- Eat more raw, unprocessed foods.

- Clear the junk food out of your pantry and throw it all away. (Donate unopened and fresh packages to your local food bank.)

- Use slow cooking methods when possible.

- Avoid eating barbecued food all summer long.

- Take the time to read nutrition labels. After a short while, you'll know in a glance what foods have the optimal nutrition, which have hidden sugars, and which should be avoided.

- Avoid sugar and sugary foods wherever possible.

- Add anti-oxidants to your daily food and water intake.

- Avoid artificial sweeteners, especially diet soda—they can make you crave sugary foods even more.

- Take a multivitamin and mineral supplement every day.

- Keep your hands busy (knitting, drawing, cracking walnuts!) when you feel the urge to put something in your mouth.

- Spend a minute thinking about what you want to put into your body *before* you put it in!

- If you're craving something sweet, set the timer for 10 minutes and see if the craving passes. Chances are, it will. Then you can have a healthy snack and drink a refreshing glass of water.

PART II

All About
Treatments

4

Treatment Glossary

THIS CHAPTER WILL COVER all the basics you'll need to know about the products and procedures I'd recommend for your anti-aging concerns. It starts with the least invasive and least expensive (over-the-counter products available without a prescription), then moves on to prescription-only treatments and procedures that target deeper layers of the skin, with longer-lasting results (and, of course, more potential for side effects). These more intensive treatments should be performed only in an experienced dermatologist's office.

Once you familiarize yourself with these treatments and procedures, you can make an informed decision about which products or treatments interest you and which may be best for your individual needs. Then you can go to the detailed chapters in part III to apply this knowledge to the specific areas of concern.

In each section, I'll explain what the product or procedure is and what it can or cannot do. Where applicable, I'll give you a truthful look at the pain factor (often grossly understated), recuperation period, and how long the product or procedure lasts.

Treatments from Least to Most Intensive

- Over-the-Counter (OTC) Skin-Care Products
- Prescription Topicals

- Mechanical Exfoliation

- Intense Pulsed Light, GentleWaves LED, Photodynamic Therapy, Coblation, Thermage, and Titan

- Injectible Fillers

- Muscle Freezers

- Chemical Peels

- Lasers

Over-the-Counter (OTC) Skin-Care Products

These products are available without prescription. They're available in drugstores, department stores, beauty specialty stores such as Sephora, and on websites. They range in price from a few dollars to thousands of dollars.

There are several categories of OTC products for anti-aging concerns. Use of these products should be part of your regular regimen:

- Moisturizers

- Anti-aging creams

- Wrinkle relaxers and smoothers

- Eye creams

- Microdermabrasion and peels

- Sunscreens (covered in chapter 2)

There are also products that target more specific needs. They will be covered in the chapters in part III, as noted:

- Whiteners (covered in chapter 6)

- Pore treatments (covered in chapter 8)

- Redness/rosacea treatments (covered in chapter 20)

Fredric Brandt, MD

MOISTURIZERS

A moisturizer is a cream, lotion, serum, or ointment designed to increase the hydration of your skin. Your skin changes over time, so your need to hydrate it will change, too. If your skin is dry or flaky, or irritated and red (due to seborrheic dermatitis, which I'll discuss on page 154), it likely needs moisture. Even if you have oily skin, you still need to protect the skin's outer layers from daily assaults from irritants, so a moisturizer will be the most basic weapon in your anti-aging arsenal.

There are three different types of ingredients in moisturizers: occlusive, humectant, or emollient.

An *occlusive* moisturizer is meant to prevent the evaporation, or transepidermal water loss, from the skin. It does this by forming a barrier with an emollient ingredient, such as mineral oil, beeswax, paraffin, silicones, petrolatum, lanolin, squalane, shea butter, or a natural oil like almond or jojoba.

Most occlusive moisturizers tend to be heavy and oil-based. Vaseline is a good example of this.

A *humectant* moisturizer attracts water so it can remain on the skin's surface; it can pull it from the deeper layers of the skin or from the environment. Ingredients that do this include hyaluronic acid, alpha hydroxy acids, sorbitol, glycerin, propylene glycol, urea, and sodium lactate.

The best kind of moisturizers use *emollients*, substances that fill in the spaces between skin cells to smooth them out. Emollients, such as lanolin, sodium hyaluronate, glycerine, and glycerl stearate, can have both occlusive and humectant properties.

Moisturizers are *not* drugs, and no claims can be made that "prove" that they *are* as effective as drugs. Choose products you like depending on texture, scent, and how they make you feel. Remember that the priciest is not always the best.

What Can a Moisturizer Do? Moisturizers have a very simple function: they treat dry skin, by bringing moisture to it. By hydrating the skin and coating its outer layers, you will plump it up and make some of the lines look less visible. One of the most common ingredients, for instance, is hyaluronic acid, which by nature attracts water to it. (When injected, hyaluronic acid is a volume replacer—so don't get confused when you see it on the label.)

What Can't a Moisturizer Do? A moisturizer by definition *cannot* treat wrinkles. All it can do is lock in moisture.

Be very wary of any moisturizer making specific anti-wrinkle claims. Moisturizers should smooth skin, and by doing so, skin may *seem* to be less wrinkled. But this is a temporary effect and will quickly wear off.

How Often Should I Use Moisturizer? First, you need to determine your skin type. Are you oily, oily only or primarily in the T-zone (area around your forehead and cheeks), oily in some spots and dry in others (which is combination skin), or dry all over?

As we age, our skin naturally loses moisture, so most women who come to me with aging concerns have dry or normal skin. If your skin is dry or normal, you should moisturize in the morning and at night. Those with dry skin can use a heavier night cream. (The biggest difference between day and night creams is that night creams tend be more occlusive and do not contain sunscreen.) You don't need to use creams more often than that, as you can cause breakouts and irritation. Be sure to keep the air in your home or office hydrated with humidifiers if you live or work in a dry environment.

If your skin is combination, feel free to use different products. Use a lighter moisturizer, or none at all, on the oily areas, and a richer one on the dry areas.

Oily skin can benefit from a lightweight moisturizer, to hold in water.

If you have very oily skin, believe it or not, you'll still need to hydrate it with the most lightweight moisturizer you like, at least at night. As you should be using a sunscreen, that should take care of hydration during the day. Don't forget a bit of eye cream, as the skin around the eye area is thinner and more prone to dryness even in those with oily skin.

ANTI-AGING/WRINKLE CREAMS

The anti-aging market is booming, and not just for boomers. It's big, big business for cosmetics companies, because, well, who wants to look old?

There are literally thousands of anti-aging creams available, and by the time you read this sentence, another one has probably been launched. What the expensive creams have is nicer packaging and lavish advertising campaigns to back up their often specious claims.

What drives me crazy is the pseudo-science used to sell a lot of these wrinkle creams. Ads will trumpet "30 percent improvement!" Well, improvement from what, and in whom? What consumers saw was not what was measured. Was this a rigorously controlled, double-blind study as mandated by the FDA for drugs, or an in-house survey of ten employee testers? It can be extremely confusing and frustrating for consumers to understand what can or cannot work effectively when it comes to anti-aging creams. There are some terrific OTC products that will give visible results if used regularly over a period of one to two months. There are others that are hyped with extravagant claims yet are little better than expensive snake oil.

Bear in mind that the only skin-care products that have been studied for safety and effectiveness, and are approved by the FDA to treat aging skin, are tretinoin creams, such as Renova or Tazorac. These are prescription creams and not available OTC.

In other words, there is no OTC anti-wrinkle cream that can legitimately claim to be scientifically proven and FDA approved to treat wrinkles. Clear on that one?

What you can buy OTC are what's called *cosmeceuticals.* Cosmeceuticals fall into that gray area between a product with no active ingredients (like plain old mineral oil) and a prescription drug that must be regulated by the FDA. According to the FDA, cosmetics are classified as inert substances "intended to be rubbed, poured, sprinkled, or sprayed on, introduced into, or otherwise applied to the human body . . . for cleansing, beautifying, promoting attractiveness, or altering the appearance." This category includes skin moisturizers, perfumes, lipsticks, fingernail polishes, eye and facial makeup preparations, shampoos, permanent waves, hair colors, toothpastes, and deodorants, as well as any material intended for use as a component of a cosmetic product.

A drug, on the other hand, is defined by the FDA as a substance "intended for use in the diagnosis, cure, mitigation, treatment, or prevention of disease, and articles (other than food) intended to affect the structure or any function of the body of man or other animals."

The FDA doesn't recognize the cosmeceutical category, and this is where the extravagant claims come in. Although cosmeceuticals are not drugs, they can include ingredients that do really work. The difference is that manufacturers cannot claim that the cosmeceutical product in any way alters the structure or function of the skin. So you'll see ads that say "may reduce" or "helps reduce the appearance of fine lines." Any claims more specific than that, such as "effectively repairs the skin," would change the classification from unregulated OTC cosmeceutical to FDA-regulated drug—one with mandated, rigorously controlled studies that take years and countless millions of dollars to perform.

Another warning bell are the claims that "83 percent of those tested saw visible changes" or "46 percent improvement in only two weeks," and so on. You have no way of knowing whether the control group consisted of five or five hundred testers, and just how "visible" those changes really were.

When considering which anti-aging product to buy, you want to look for ingredients that have been thoroughly researched and have a proven track record of effectiveness and safety. There have been, for example, many studies on the effectiveness of retinols on collagen stimulation. There have been many other studies on anti-oxidants such as green tea. You also need to buy from reputable companies that do not make overinflated claims, especially since the cosmetic industry is so loosely regulated and prone to hype. You should be able to contact them and ask what percentage of the active ingredients trumpeted in their ads are used in their product, especially in comparison to the averages used in other products, and ask who does the testing to ensure that the level claimed is the level in the box. (Vitamins are often found to have the dosage level far under what's claimed on the box when tested by a neutral third party.)

Recently, some anti-aging creams costing thousands of dollars have come on the market. I suggest you save the money you've earmarked for the super-expensive Goo of the Month and use it to pay for a consultation with a qualified cosmetic dermatologist instead. (Sometimes, I'm shocked to say, a small jar of the Goo of the Month will cost more than several months of consultations!) Of course, it's totally up to you to find the right skin-care plan, and buying this book is the right step in evaluating all your options.

Frankly, although top-quality ingredients and the rigorous control needed to oversee their manufacture definitely cost money, there are in my opinion no

Fredric Brandt, MD

ingredients that warrant a $1,000+ price tag on a jar of cream. There's always the placebo factor, of course—thinking that because a cream is so expensive it simply has to work more effectively. Or the pleasure factor—knowing that you can afford such a luxury and showing off the beautiful packaging.

There is, obviously, a difference between a $10 drugstore cream and a $100 dermatologist-created cream. A less expensive product will not have the glossy packaging and the heavy glass bottle with a gold top. It will also not have active ingredients, with the same *purity* or concentration. But is a $1,000 cream 100 times better than a $10 cream? What do you think?

And could you go to a dermatologist instead for much longer lasting wrinkle treatments? Yes, you can. Caveat emptor!

What Should an Anti-Aging Cream Do? An anti-aging cream, in theory, should diminish fine lines and wrinkles. It should firm the skin and increase your skin's elasticity. It should even out your skin tone and texture. It should also help prevent collagen breakdown and help stimulate the growth of new collagen.

Not every anti-aging cream will have all these properties, but whatever you choose to use in your regimen should be effectively tackling these concerns.

What Can't an Anti-Aging Cream Do? They can't totally eliminate severe wrinkles, creases, and folds, but they can soften their appearance. No OTC cream can completely replace lost volume in the face.

Some anti-aging products in the form of serums are, depending on whom you ask, seen as more concentrated formulas to their cream counterparts. But again, as the cosmetics/aesthetics of the product are so important (to be lightweight, not sticky, penetrate quickly, and look translucent), sometimes the formulations might not be as potent as consumers think they are, especially since there are ingredients that are by nature not translucent, or need the "help" of other ingredients to penetrate the skin. It's best to regard serums as a nice way to complement your regimen and give it a boost, but they are not replacements for moisturizers or anti-aging creams.

How Often Should I Use an Anti-Aging Cream? Every day. Morning or night. Whatever you choose, use sparingly and follow directions. Glopping on a lot of cream can cause breakouts and will not diminish more wrinkles. Day creams tend to be lighter, as they are intended for use under makeup, and they often contain sunscreen (although not enough sunscreen to provide the broad-spectrum protection that you need). Night creams tend to be richer and thicker, with no SPF.

The OTC products for anti-aging fall into several categories:

- Alpha hydroxy acids

- Anti-oxidants

- Collagen promoters/retinols

- Peptide creams

- Microdermabrasion

- Home peels

Alpha Hydroxy Acids (AHAs) and Beta Hydroxy Acids (BHAs) Say "acid" and many people think "burn." Well, you can forget about this concept and instead embrace the wide variety of acid products, as they have an intrinsic ability to exfoliate and smooth the outermost layer of skin and speed up the skin-cell turnover that naturally diminishes with age. As natural chemical exfoliators, they allow the dead skin cells on the surface of your skin (the stratum corneum) to be sloughed off properly, revealing fresh new skin underneath.

Nefertiti was a big fan of exfoliation back in her day, washing herself every morning with a mixture of water and natural lime water, rubbing her body with a clay paste made from Nile mud, and rubbing away rough spots on her body with pumice. She often followed that exfoliation with ostrich-egg, clay, oil, and milk masks. Fast-forward a few centuries, and women used milk baths or lemon juice as the basis for at-home skin treatments. They didn't know that what helped refresh their skin were the hydroxy acids found inside—they just knew that these liquids had visible effects.

Alpha hydroxy acids are water-soluble and come from many sources. Glycolic, in concentrations of 2 percent to 20 percent, are made from sugar cane; citric, from citrus fruits; lactic, from sour milk; malic, from apples; phytic, from rice; and tartaric, from grapes. Beta hydroxy acids (salicylic, from willow bark and sweet birch trees) are oil-soluble. Glycolic acid is the most commonly used AHA, because it's the most effective, but it's also the most irritating. Salicylic acid, which is soluble in fats, can also penetrate into the gunk clogging up pores, so it's great for oily skin.

AHA creams can also boost collagen production, which helps diminish fine wrinkles and other signs of aging or sun-damaged skin. They can help fade brown spots (hyperpigmentation) and smooth the skin's top surface.

Use of any AHAs causes greater sensitivity to the sun, so you must protect yourself with sunscreen and hats, and avoid sun exposure altogether whenever possible if you apply these products.

Most OTC products contain about 4 percent to 8 percent active AHA, if that. Since the FDA doesn't mandate the disclosure of AHA concentration in OTC products, chances are high you won't know what you're getting. (This is complicated by the fact that the pH, or the acid balance, in a cream, will determine the amount of free acid that is available to do the job.) The only way to do so is with a reputable company that lists the ingredients in detail, or move on to nonprescription formulations sold in dermatologists' offices or prescription-strength creams and peels.

Nearly everyone can use a low-strength, over-the-counter AHA cream every day. Remember that although AHA creams feel like moisturizers, they are treatment creams. If you apply an AHA cream in the morning, the correct application order is AHA cream, then moisturizer, then sunscreen.

Anti-Oxidants Anti-oxidants are substances that fight free radicals. As I described in earlier chapters, free radicals are a highly reactive oxygen species, imbalanced molecules that try to steal electrons from healthy cells to neutralize their own charge. Produced inside our bodies and by the outside environment, free radicals cause damage that results in premature aging.

An anti-oxidant cream is a protective cream designed to prevent the free radicals from doing their dirty work. This can be done with chemicals that block the reaction, or with substances, such as the tiny spheres called fullerenes that, instead of merely blocking the chemical reaction, can actually scavenge up the free radicals and neutralize them.

64

10 MINUTES / 10 YEARS

Commonly used anti-oxidant ingredients found in OTC products are: grapeseed extract, green tea, pomegranate, and vitamins E and C. One of the most potent of these is green tea. Its active compound, epigallocatechin gallate (EGCG), is more than 100 times more effective at neutralizing free radicals than is vitamin C.

Collagen Promoters/Retinols Collagen promoters are creams that send signals to the skin to stimulate collagen production.

Collagen, as you know by now, is a protein that is the building block of connective tissue. It's actually a string of complex molecules, so it can't penetrate through the surface of the skin and bind to your internal collagen when applied in the form of a topical product. Therefore, the collagen in an OTC cream is a great moisturizing agent, but it will remain on the surface.

Retinoids, or tretinoin, on the other hand, are a modified form of vitamin A acids that do penetrate the skin to stimulate cellular regeneration and collagen production. They can also improve skin texture and clarity, reduce brown spots (hyperpigmentation), minimize pore size, and diminish fine wrinkles. As such they are classified as a drug and are only available by prescription. The reason I mention them here is that the OTC version of retinoids are called retinols, and they are available without a prescription. The big advantage is that prescription retinoids can cause skin irritation, and the much smaller concentration permissible in OTC retinol creams makes them less prone to cause redness.

Even though OTC retinols do contain such a small amount of the active ingredients allowed in their preparation, using them will still help promote collagen stimulation. Be aware, though, that the concentration of active retinol must be high enough, usually 0.04 percent to 0.07 percent, to make any kind of real difference in your skin. If a skin cream doesn't formulate the retinol delivery system properly, you'll be throwing away your money.

For those whose skin is easily irritated by prescription retinoids or stronger AHAs, OTC retinols are a good solution. They are converted to retinoic acid in the skin, albeit without the same potency as the retinoids can be. It's like running a race. It may take you a little longer to get to the finish line with retinols, but you're still going to get the results.

There are also creams that inhibit the breakdown of collagen, called collagenase inhibitors, or matrix metallo-proteinases (MMP) inhibitors. (MMP is the enzyme that causes the breakdown of collagen.)

As with AHAs, retinols make the skin far more susceptible to sun damage, so use of sunscreen with them is a must.

Peptide Creams A peptide is a fragment of a protein. A protein is made up of amino acids. Amino acids link together to form peptides; bigger groups are called polypeptides, which form proteins such as collagen. Certain peptide combinations are able to act as cell regulators to tell certain processes to be turned on or off. They're little messengers that tell the body what to do. In skincare creams, the peptides may help with the production of collagen, as well as relax the muscles that cause wrinkles.

However, as you'll see in the next section, no topical cream made by any company can ever equal the effect of an injected product.

HOW TO DECODE A LABEL

My patients often tell me how confused they are by the information on the back of a jar of cream. Many of the ingredients have long, complicated, and bizarre-sounding chemical names. How can you tell what they mean, and what their purpose is?

First of all, if there are any active ingredients that are classified as drugs, they will be listed at the top. If you look at a bottle of sunscreen, you'll see chemicals such as avobenzone and octinoxate listed at the top, along with their percentages. Below them, the inactive ingredients will be listed. If there are no separate active/inactive listings, then no ingredient in this specific product has been classified as a drug by the FDA.

Ingredients are listed in descending order of quantity, from highest to lowest. Usually, the first ingredient is water (aqua). What's confusing is that the concentration might be skewed. Let's say one ingredient is super-potent, and therefore is listed near the bottom, because only a tiny amount is needed to be effective. There's no way for the average consumer to know when less actually might mean more. What you can do is use common sense. If a company is hyping an active ingredient on the front of the box, yet this active ingredient is at the bottom of the ingredient list, my hype alert would go into overdrive. But on the other hand, some ingredients are effective at a 1 percent concentration. The overall balance and composition of the cream, as well as the vehicle substance used to transport the ingredient, will affect how this percentage is delivered too.

In addition, many companies make their claims based on the ingredients as they've been tested in the *laboratory*. The properties of the ingredient *change* once you put it in a cream, so it might not necessarily do in real life what the chemical lab says it does in the test tube. And you can't know if this lab-created ingredient might change or become completely ineffective once it's combined with other ingredients.

Tough regulations in the United States and in foreign markets also mean manufacturers must split certain raw materials or certain ingredients into parts, leading to what's labeled as a fragmented formulation. To make things even more complicated, many ingredients can be in the form of solutions or blends, and from that, the ingredients listed may actually have been split into two or three parts of the formula. This makes it next to impossible to decipher the true—and truly active—composition of the product.

Nor must a label tell you the source of the ingredient or what kind of quality control is in place by the manufacturer. Take green tea. There are thousands of suppliers, with different qualities of active ingredients, which is why you should try to buy the best creams you can afford, from reliable companies. The percentage listed for a certain ingredient might be the same with a $6.99 cream as a $69.99 cream, but that doesn't mean you can make a blanket assumption that these creams will work in an identical fashion.

Consumers who read articles online or in women's magazines have worries about certain ingredients. For instance, they'll claim that manufacturers talk a lot about using natural ingredients, so why are there chemical preservatives in their product? The answer is simple: Without preservatives, no product would have a shelf life longer than a week or two. It would become rancid and spoiled. It could harm you.

Or, with the preservatives called parabens, there have been studies where traces have been found in tissue taken from women with breast cancer. Consumers will read that and make the unwarranted assumption that parabens cause breast cancer. In reality, parabens are the most studied and used cosmetic preservative in the world, with the best safety record. After rumors went flying on the internet, the European Commission and the French authorities released a document stating that parabens are safe and the rumors are not correct. Ironically, products that are paraben-free may contain ingredients that don't have the same safety record as parabens.

Consumers also worry about allergies. Among the most common allergens in cosmetic products are fragrances. Many brands use only natural oils, not perfumes, such as citrus and lavender, to scent their products. (Face creams need to have some sort of fragrance or they'd smell unpleasantly of fat.) All U.S. manufacturers must test their products for allergic reactions. The test used is called a Repeat Insult Patch Test (RIPT). It's important to realize that consumers will often attribute a reaction to a product to an "allergy," but in reality it could have been caused by any number of factors, such as diet, an interaction between different products, or failure to follow directions (such as using too much or not using sunscreen for products that are photo-reactive).

Consumers also have misconceptions about other ingredients. One in particular is urea. I think people see that word and think *urine*. In fact, urea is an effective moisturizing agent. Or squalane. Some people think it's derived from fish, which it can be, but it's also derived from olive oil.

Bottom line: Be an educated consumer. If you have questions about a product, call the company. Don't be afraid to ask. If you have reactions to the product, return it. (Again, your reaction may be caused by other factors, unless you have an immediate reaction the instant you apply the product.) You should be given a full refund. But you should also follow directions. Using too much of any product can cause irritation and breakouts.

WRINKLE RELAXERS AND SMOOTHERS

This category covers the type of creams that are specifically applied to wrinkles to minimize their appearance. Ever since the manufacturers of StriVectin posed the question "Better than Botox?"—which, I must say, is absolutely genius marketing—consumers have flocked to try it and see for themselves.

68

What Can a Wrinkle Relaxer Do? An anti-wrinkle cream is an adjunct product to be used along with moisturizers or anti-aging creams. It should contain ingredients, such as amino acids, peptides, and soothing botanicals, that calm and relax the skin. Effects can last up to eight to ten hours. If used daily, wrinkle creams should have a cumulative effect after about two weeks of regular use.

Be sure to apply wrinkle relaxer by *patting*, not rubbing or spreading, gently on expression lines, such as those found around the eyes, between the brows, on the forehead, around the lips, and on the neck. Always apply a wrinkle relaxer to clean skin, before applying any moisturizers. Otherwise you'll just be wasting your time and money. Wait two minutes, then follow with your regular anti-aging cream and sunscreen.

Another form of wrinkle relaxer is a smoother or primer. These are treatment creams that usually contain silicone and give a smooth finish to the skin, thereby diminishing wrinkles. They can also contain ingredients that will help stimulate collagen production.

What Can't a Wrinkle Relaxer Do? Permanently fill in wrinkles. They work best on superficial wrinkles, for a short period of time. They will have a mild effect on moderate to deep wrinkles or folds.

Bottom line: There is no topical wrinkle cream that is better than Botox!

How Often Should I Use a Wrinkle Relaxer? Every day, morning and/or night, as needed.

EYE CREAMS

The eye area is often neglected when in truth it needs more than an extra boost. The skin around the eyes has fewer oil glands than the rest of the face, so it becomes drier more quickly. It also is prone to fine wrinkles that can progress into full-blown crow's-feet. Bags and sags can make skin look crepey and mottled. Visible blood vessels create dark circles. Not a charming sight.

Eye creams tend to be thicker than regular moisturizers, so use sparingly. A little goes a long way. Eye creams also have been ophthalmologist tested, so they will not cause the same kind of stinging or burning if you accidentally rub some into your eyes as would a regular moisturizer. Their gentleness makes them ideal for sensitive skin.

My patients often ask if they really do need a separate eye cream, or if it's just hype. I tell them that yes, they do need an eye cream. Make it a habit to gently pat on a good eye cream and follow that with a sunscreen every morning. Use it again, sans the sunscreen, at night to keep the squints and lines at bay.

I'll discuss more about eye creams, dark circles, and puffiness in chapter 10.

How Often Should I Use an Eye Cream? Every day. Morning and night.

CHOOSING THE RIGHT CLEANSER

Believe it or not, there is such a thing as too clean when it comes to skin. I've treated many overzealous cleansers who figure that if twice a day is good, then more is even better. I gently remind them that aging skin needs a gentle touch, and overdoing the need to feel "squeaky clean" strips the skin of needed oils and natural protection against the elements. Which means that the deodorant soap you use in the shower or bath is never to be applied to the face!

Some of my patients prefer to use plain old bar soap, and in that case I'm happy to recommend Dove, as it is gentle and effective. Most, however, like the ease of liquid cleansers. If your skin is dry, choose a creamy cleanser that doesn't foam; normal skin can pretty much tolerate anything; and oily skin responds best to foaming gels or liquids. Those with sensitive skin should look for soothing botanicals, such as green tea and grapeseed extract.

It's best to clean your face twice a day, but if you're running late in the morning, it's okay to skip it. Never go to bed without a thorough cleansing and removal of all makeup. It can cause breakouts on your skin and irritation in and around your eyes.

Toners aren't a mandatory part of your cleansing regimen, but they're great at restoring the skin's pH balance, and a lot of my patients like them. Avoid any with astringents, unless you have seriously oily skin, as they'll dehydrate your skin. Best for aging skin are those with AHAs and anti-oxidants.

HOME MICRODERMABRASION

Microdermabrasion is a great way to exfoliate, brightening and polishing the skin's surface. It smoothes fine lines and wrinkles, and also helps improve scars. It also allows the creams you put on afterward to penetrate more deeply into the skin.

As we age, skin cell turnover naturally slows down—from an average of twenty-eight days when in our twenties, to an average of up to fifty days in our fifties. Regular exfoliation is an important step in maintaining a healthy glow. Without it, skin can appear blotchy and dull.

Good microdermabrasion creams and pastes have tiny beads, composed of superfine mineral crystals with a slightly rough texture, that do a more intensive sloughing off of dead skin cells than a regular cream. Plus the chemical exfoliants loosen the sort of cement that binds cells together, so that outer layer of cells comes off more easily.

Be careful not to overdo it. I've seen patients who've rubbed their faces raw in their zeal to exfoliate. You don't need to rub. Even if you use your microdermabrasion paste at night, you must use sunscreen the next morning (as well as *every* morning!), as your skin will be much more sensitive to the sun following a treatment.

Some companies are now offering handheld microdermabrasion devices that they claim will speed up exfoliation. I don't recommend them, as the potential for serious irritation is just too great in inexperienced hands. I've seen far too many patients with bright red, peeling faces that were a little too zealous in their regimens.

Basically, think of microdermabrasion as a sort of skin polishing. It should be a regular part of your skin-care routine, especially if you can't get to see a dermatologist. Just not a *daily* part!

How Often Should I Do Microdermabrasion? Try starting off with once a week, see how your skin tolerates the product, then work up to two or three times a week. Find the right balance. Gently massage the cream onto the skin. Do not rub. And don't overdo it, as you can cause some serious redness, flaking, and dryness.

Fredric Brandt, MD

NONPRESCRIPTION MD PRODUCTS

Dermatologists often offer products with the same ingredients as OTC creams, but in more potent concentrations. As such, there is a greater potential for side effects, but you'll be monitored by your dermatologist, who can tweak the formula or regimen till it's optimal for you. Two of the most popular lines are M.D. Forté and SkinMedica.

Do bear in mind, however, that many dermatologists buy the same nonprescription products from the same suppliers and have them labeled with their own names. (This is called private labeling.) There's nothing wrong with this, as the products are quality-controlled. And because they are doctor-controlled and sold, you shouldn't have to worry about any of the exaggerated or downright false claims you might encounter at the cosmetic counters in department stores or on websites. As your dermatologist will have examined your skin prior to selling them, the results will be more realistically tailored to your specific needs. And if there are any questions or side effects, your doctor can help you.

Most of the nonprescription MD products are creams and peels, with a higher concentration of the acid component. Take glycolic acid. How well it works depends on its concentration as well as its pH balance. So a higher, MD-only concentration of 10 percent doesn't necessarily tell the whole story. Something with a low pH at 5 percent can actually be more potent than something with a high pH at 10 percent. Ideally, your dermatologist will know your skin type and sensitivity predisposition, and give you the right formula. Or she might start you with a milder peel, follow your progress, and then as you become more tolerant, increase the level of strength. Usually, glycolic acid products can range from 10 percent up to over 30 percent. Start slow and work your way up to a stronger concentration, if needed. If you jump right into a strong concentration, your skin can get irritated.

Prevage, the idebenol anti-oxidant cream made by Allergan (which also makes Botox), used to be sold entirely through MD offices. Now it's available in a lower strength by Elizabeth Arden. I find this a bit perplexing. Why would you buy a half-strength product in a department store if you can get a full-strength version at the doctor's office?

Nonprescription MD products are well tested and should preclude any worries about the correct dosage or potential irritants, as your dermatologist will have evaluated your skin prior to dispensing them. They're best when combined with topical prescriptions and/or procedures—which is why you've gone to see the dermatologist in the first place.

HOME PEELS

A peel done in the comfort of your home will exfoliate a superficial amount of skin cells. They can also help clear clogged pores, improve skin clarity and texture, and diminish brown spots.

Home peels are usually AHA-based, with lactic, glycolic, or other acids. Some also include anti-oxidants. These dual-purpose peels will not only exfoliate and brighten, but serve as a vehicle delivery for anti-oxidants.

A home peel can't provide the same punch as a deeper peel done by a dermatologist, but as with the retinoids/retinols, it is much less likely to cause any irritation. Start at a small area on the side of your face, to make sure you don't feel anything burning, before applying to your entire face. The goal is *not* to turn red, get crusty, blister, or peel your skin right off!

How Often Should I Do a Home Peel? Different peels can be used with different frequency; the lower the acid, the more often you can try them. It will also depend on your skin type. In general, most people can use a home peel once a week—but *never* on the same day you use any other exfoliating product (e.g., microdermabrasion). Those with very oily skin and acne may be able to tolerate a peel twice a week, whereas those with sensitive skin might only want to use one once a month.

Prescription Topicals

Prescription topicals are an easy, painless way to improve aging skin. As I've said, the only ingredient approved by the FDA to combat wrinkles are the retinoids. Nearly everyone I treat can benefit from their use.

WHAT TO LOOK FOR IN A COSMETIC DERMATOLOGIST

A good cosmetic dermatologist will evaluate your skin, discuss your options, tell you which products will work the best for your individual skin needs and which products won't, and save you not only thousands of dollars in the long run, but help you improve your skin with the use of tested and effective ingredients and procedures.

I tell my patients that they brush their teeth at home, but that can't fix a chipped tooth. Skin care is no different.

All cosmetic dermatologists have the same tools—access to the same studies, the same prescription products, the same vials of injectibles, and the same laser machines. But the question is, Who's using them on your face?

Your treatment will only be as good as the hand wielding it.

You can see evidence of this in every women's magazine, full of photographs of celebrities with lips puffed up to exaggerated proportions (unaffectionately known as "trout pout") or foreheads so unnaturally smooth and devoid of lines that you could practically go ice skating on them. *Someone* had to have provided these treatments. Frankly, any good dermatologist needs to know when to say no. Or to tell patients that the look they're requesting is not feasible, practical, or something you'd recommend for their particular anatomy (such as a sixty-five-year-old with thin lips asking for Angelina Jolie's smackers).

First, be an educated consumer and do your homework prior to making an appointment, especially if you're considering having any advanced procedures done involving needles, lasers, or peeling. All treatments have risks, as small as they may be (if they happen to you, they're not small at all). Complications can happen. You want to make sure you're in experienced hands, just to be on the safe side.

I would not recommend that you go to a facialist for in-depth skin-care advice or treatments. Their facials might be soothing, but their advice is often wrong. This can be dangerous, for example, if you're getting acid peels and they mix up the wrong concentration. It's better, of course, if a facial is done in a dermatologist's office where there is interaction between the physician and the esthetician to create a plan for the patient. So, by all means, have facials if you like them and you feel they help your skin. But don't use facialists who are not physicians for any sort of more complicated treatments, and regard their recommendations about products with a healthy dose of skepticism.

Another must to avoid are those who go around the country performing at "injectibles parties." I think it's ludicrous that anyone would remotely consider being injected by a stranger in someone else's home, just to save money. You have no idea if the person wielding the needle is ethical or even has any medical training. You have no idea what's actually in the syringe, whether the product is legitimate, watered-down, or sterile. It's a recipe for disaster, yet my patients are always gossiping about who flew in whom to do the deed in Mrs. So-and-So's house. I can't tell you how many times I've seen patients with lumps in their faces, who need drastic correction to undo the damage. It's absolutely crazy what some people will allow to be injected into their faces! I hope you're not going to be one of them.

As for physicians, well, anyone with a medical license can perform any medical procedure. Plastic surgeons can do face-lifts and Restylane injections. Would you ask your obstetrician to give you Botox, or would you ask your dermatologist to deliver your baby?

For cosmetic procedures, you should see a cosmetic dermatologist who specializes in those treatments. Some dermatologists concentrate on skin cancers or acne, for instance. Ask before your make an appointment.

Before you see the doctor, you can also ask to see before and after photographs. Even if the quality isn't great, such as with Polaroids, it's better to ask and get an idea of the results. This helps you have more realistic expectations, and it also will give you an idea of the doctor's technique. Some doctors have a more heavy hand than others. Some are quite subtle. If you want subtle, don't choose a doctor with a reputation for over-the-top results.

You should ask all of these questions and be satisfied with the answers prior to any treatments.

Is the doctor trained in dermatology? Is he or she board certified in a specialty? (Board certification provides additional training.)

Has this dermatologist had additional specialized training in these procedures as well? If so, when and where? After all, there are so many technological advances of late, you need to know that your doctor is up to date and not relying on techniques or materials that are verging on the obsolete.

Are the treatments you're interested in the primary focus of this dermatologist? Some are better trained or prefer to use lasers than injectibles, for instance. You won't know unless you ask.

What kind of results are to be expected?

How many treatments are needed, on average?

How often must I see the dermatologist for maintenance? What will happen if these appointments are postponed or skipped?

Are there any side effects? Could I be allergic to any of the compounds used? (*Always* tell your dermatologist of any known allergies prior to any treatment.) If there is bruising, peeling, swelling, irritation, or bleeding, how long might it last? Can you go back to work afterward?

What is the pain factor? I have patients who like to joke that whenever a doctor says, "You'll just feel a little pinch," it means they'll really be screaming off the table. Ask for a realistic description of what the pain might be. Ask what numbing agents and anesthesia are used. Tell the doctor if you're needle-phobic!

What is the cost? Are there hidden fees? Are there extended payment plans, or discounts for paying up front (with treatments that involve multiple visits, for example). Will insurance cover any of these treatments? (That's unlikely if they're cosmetic.)

And then there's the dermatologist's bedside manner. Sometimes you might be happy with the results, but you just don't click with your dermatologist, personality-wise. The doctor might be brusque, or too talkative, or too slow to return phone calls. As aging is an ongoing concern, and you will hopefully be seeing your dermatologist over many years, it's crucial to establish a good relationship and rapport. If you're not happy, walk away with a copy of your records and find someone who's a better fit.

RETINOIDS

Retinoids are vitamin A derivatives that form the front line of defense for anyone who's not quite ready or willing to use injectible fillers or other dermatologist treatments. They do work. They take but a minute to apply. But there is a huge downside: they can cause serious irritation, especially if there is sun exposure. Anyone choosing to use a retinoid must also commit to use of daily sunscreen and repeated application of sunscreen whenever outside. All day. Every day.

What Can Retinoids Do? Retinoids, or tretinoin, stimulate collagen production. They can reduce wrinkles and other signs of aging, such as brown spots and pore size. They can also effectively treat adult acne. Retinoids are vitamin A derivatives that increase collagen synthesis and help reduce both chronological aging and photo-aging. Renova and Retin-A, with the active ingredient tretinoin, have been proven to help diminish fine-line wrinkling and polish the surface of the skin. Tretinoin and tazarotene, the active component of Tazorac, are the *only* skin-care ingredients that are approved by the FDA for the treatment of fine wrinkles.

I often prescribe Renova in addition to using injectibles. Even the best fillers wear off over time. Aging happens. No one treatment lasts forever!

As retinoids can cause irritation at first, usually in the form of redness and flakiness, discuss how best to minimize any reactions with your dermatologist. There are different formulations, such as gels and creams, in different concentrations.

When you do use a retinoid, daily sunscreen is an absolute must, as retinoids make you extremely susceptible to sunburn. For some of my patients, getting a terrible, peeling burn on their faces because they "forgot" to put on their sunscreen yet again is the only way to make them realize how badly they abuse their skin and how they need to protect it more than ever. The most popular and strongest retinoid is Avage, also known as Tazorac. (Tazorac is usually prescribed for psoriasis and acne. Avage is identical, but the insurance companies in their infinite wisdom decided it needed to be renamed, as otherwise those with legitimate medical problems such as psoriasis would not be reimbursed for a prescription that also has cosmetic applications.) Other retinoids are Differin (adapalene) and Renova (Retin-A) (both tretinoin). They're all slightly different, as they affect different retinoid receptors.

Retinoids come in various formulations and strengths, depending on your skin type. If your skin is oily, a gel might be best; normal skin can tolerate the creams; and those with sensitive skin will probably be given Renova. Your dermatologist will decide what will work best for you and monitor your skin's response. Over time, irritation and redness will lessen. But the need for sunscreen will not!

What Can't Retinoids Do? Retinoids can't treat moderate to deep wrinkles or creases. They can't replace lost volume. They can't fix sagging skin.

How Often Should I Use a Retinoid? Every day. Your dermatologist will decide on the strength and on whether to use the retinoid once or twice a day. I usually advise patients to apply it every other night at first. It's often hard for patients to stick with the program, because they're annoyed by the perfectly normal irritation triggered by retinoids—even though it means the retinoid is working. Be patient. Expect to see results in approximately three months.

Always apply only to dry skin. Retinoids cause more irritation if applied to damp or wet skin.

Mechanical Exfoliation

MICRODERMABRASION

Mechanical exfoliation, or microdermabrasion, involves the use of a device that first sprays mineral crystals onto the skin and then sucks them back up inside. It's like sandblasting the skin. As the crystals are swooshed back up into the vacuum, the dead outer layers of skin go with them.

There are many different types of microdermabrasion systems available. Most of them use aluminum oxide, sodium bicarbonate (salt), or diamond crystals. The intensity is controlled by the volume of the crystals emitted as well as the intensity of the vacuum suction. It's always better to start slow, gradually increase the intensity—and not overdo it!

What Can Microdermabrasion Do? Microdermabrasion is the equivalent of a superficial acid peel. It's a terrific way to exfoliate, improve skin texture, unblock pores, remove excess oil, and reduce fine, superficial wrinkles.

What Can't Microdermabrasion Do? Microdermabrasion has a slow, cumulative effect. One treatment will not do much of anything except give you a glow.

Be sure to remember that microdermabrasion will be a total waste of your time and money if you go out in the sun without adequate protection afterward—and not just after the procedure, but *every* day. All the wrinkles and hyperpigmentation spots will come right back.

How Often Should I Get Microdermabrasion? You'll need up to eight sessions, spaced one to two weeks apart for optimal results. This can be repeated every year, as needed.

Pain Factor There should be no pain. If there is any pain, ask for the settings to be lowered.

Recuperation You'll be slightly pink afterward, as if you'd gotten a sunburn. Treat this with a good moisturizer and makeup. Be sure to avoid the sun.

DERMABRASION

Unlike microdermabrasion, dermabrasion is a heavy-duty procedure. Dermabrasion is a mechanical means of providing deep exfoliation, reaching down into living skin cells. It's done with a wheel studded with diamond particles to abrade the skin.

I used to perform dermabrasion on many patients, with terrific results, but as this procedure has been replaced by lasers and peels, it's rarely performed anymore. Although the process itself wasn't that painful, because we'd use a freezer to numb the skin, afterward skin would be raw and crusty.

If dermabrasion is done correctly, the results can be long-lasting and spectacular, well worth the pain and lingering redness (sometimes persisting for several months). If it isn't, you are in serious, serious trouble.

You need to weigh the pros and cons carefully before considering dermabrasion. It requires a high level of technical skill, and it's become a bit of a lost art. For that reason, I don't recommend the procedure anymore, simply because a dermatologist needs many years of experience to perform it properly. If you need deep exfoliation, I suggest you stick to peels and lasers with dermatologists skilled in their use.

Intense Pulsed Light (IPL), GentleWaves LED, Photodynamic Therapy (PDT), Coblation, Thermage, and Titan

INTENSE PULSED LIGHT

Intense Pulsed Light is not a laser. It uses a multitude of wavelengths of light to stimulate collagen and lighten skin, delivered to the skin with pulses of a handheld device that flashes an intense beam of light. When pigmentation spots or red blood vessels are bombarded with the light, it's converted to heat, which is then absorbed by the body, removing the spots or redness.

The names of the procedures are different—IPL Facial, FotoFacial, PhotoFacial, Photorejuvenation, and EpiFacial—but they all basically do the same thing.

What Can IPL Do? IPL can improve skin texture, remove hyperpigmentation spots, reduce redness associated with rosacea, and treat broken blood vessels, large pores, and fine lines. It can't, however, be used on tanned skin, and those with darker skin tones are at risk for developing hyperpigmentation, hypopigmentation, and scarring.

What Can't IPL Do? IPL doesn't work on deep wrinkles. It's best for superficial wrinkles. It's most commonly used for redness and hyperpigmentation, so it's not regarded as the primary weapon against wrinkles.

How Often Should I Get IPL? Treatment is usually once a month for four months.

Pain Factor Little to none.

Recuperation Side effects should be minimal if it's done properly. Skin might be slightly red or swollen.

GENTLEWAVES LED

The GentleWaves LED light is a not a laser or an IPL. It's a photomodulation device wherein a yellow light is set at a certain wavelength. The energy from the light works on the mitochondria, the energy-producing cell organelles, to enhance rejuvenation. LED is one of the easiest treatments available and works on all skin types, even on tanned skin.

What Can LED Do? LED can prevent the breakdown of collagen, refine superficial wrinkles, help with overall skin texture, and decrease redness and inflammation. It is also useful in the treatment of sunburns.

What Can't LED Do? Take away brown spots or remove any moderate to deep wrinkles.

LED is often combined with other procedures, such as laser resurfacing, and is more effective if done right after gentle exfoliation.

How Often Should I Have LED? Each session lasts only 35 seconds; if you're treating more than one area, it'll take a few minutes. You will need to have a series of ten treatments, two or three times a week for a month or so, plus maintenance visits after that, in order to see results.

Pain Factor None.

Recuperation None.

Fredric Brandt, MD

PHOTODYNAMIC THERAPY (PDT)

Photodynamic Therapy (PDT) involves the application of Levulan Kerastick (aminolevulinic acid, or ALA, made by DUSA Pharmaceuticals, Inc.), a photo-sensitizing agent, to the skin. It's left on for up to an hour or more, then activated with IPL, blue light, or a laser, depending on the physician's choice. The heat causes a chemical reaction.

What Can PDT Do? PDT is an effective treatment for precancerous spots caused by sun damage. It also helps rejuvenate skin, shrink pores, improve texture, reduce rosacea and redness, and treat acne.

What Can't PDT Do? Treat moderate to severe wrinkles and folds. Replace lost volume.

How Often Should I Have PDT? A course of three treatments, spaced two to four weeks apart.

Pain Factor The ALA is applied without any anesthesia. It's not painful, although some patients feel a mild burning or stinging sensation. This is then removed, and depending on the light source used to activate the ALA, a topical anesthetic might be applied. Sometimes a light microdermabrasion is done prior to the application of the ALA to remove dead skin and allow better and more even penetration of the ALA.

Recuperation Skin will be red, swollen, and sore. There may be some crusting for up to a week. It is absolutely imperative to stay completely shaded from the sun for at least forty-eight hours after treatment, as any light will further activate the chemical reaction and could cause severe burning.

COBLATION (VISAGE)

During this treatment, an electrical current is passed through a saline (salt) solution to heat the skin and vaporize its top layer.

What Can Coblation Do? Treat mild to moderate wrinkles and sun damage.

What Can't Coblation Do? Treat deeper wrinkles. Replace lost volume or tighten sags.

How Often Should I Have Coblation? Once every five years, or as needed.

Pain Factor Mild to moderate. You'll need topical anesthetic cream and perhaps a painkiller prior to the procedure.

Recuperation Your skin will be sore and tender for up to a week. It will stay red for about a month.

THERMAGE

Thermage is a radio-frequency device that superheats the dermal layer of the skin, causing it to contract and as a result tighten the skin. A handheld device delivers the heat to the collagen layers while simultaneously protecting and cooling the outer layers.

What Can Thermage Do? The heat from Thermage causes an immediate contraction of collagen, followed by eventual new collagen production. It's approved by the FDA to tighten loose skin, thereby reducing wrinkles and sagging.

What Can't Thermage Do? Treat deep wrinkles. Replace lost volume.

How Often Should I Have Thermage? Every six to twelve months.

Pain Factor When Thermage was first approved, some patients reported that the pain was extremely intense. Now with new modifications, the pain is less severe, but Thermage can still hurt, especially over bony prominences. Oral prescription pain medications and/or nerve blocks and topical anesthesia are recommended.

Fredric Brandt, MD

Recuperation There is no downtime or skin irritation. Of course, if you took any prescription oral pain medication, you may need to be escorted home and should not drive.

TITAN

The Titan is a revolutionary noninvasive broad-wavelength-based infrared-emitting device made by Cutera. It emits light in the 1100 to 1800 nm wavelength range. During use, it cools the upper layers of the skin while heating up the dermis to contract the collagen fibers.

What Can Titan Do? Give you a visible tightening of lax skin, stimulate long-term collagen production, and improve skin elasticity. This will have the best effect on fine wrinkles and sagging. It's used mainly for the entire face and neck, and can also give good results for lifting the breasts, saggy abdominal skin, and saggy knee skin.

What Can't Titan Do? Treat skin texture, hyperpigmentation, or deep wrinkles. Replace lost volume.

How Often Should I Have Titan? Patients often don't see immediate results, although they may notice some feeling of a tightening in the treated area right after the procedure, which then increases for the next two to three months. Best results are seen when there are at least three treatments, spaced a month apart, and then once every year or two for maintenance. Results can last up to two years.

Pain Factor The Titan is much less painful than Thermage. Patients feel a wave of heat, but as the skin is simultaneously cooled, they rarely need any topical anesthesia.

Recuperation There is little to no downtime, as there may be some slight irritation or redness that quickly goes away.

Injectible Fillers

Fillers are the future!

As with Botox, injectible fillers have revolutionized cosmetic dermatology. The reason is simple: They treat volume loss, the aspect of intrinsic aging over which we have no control. The dimensionality in the face disappears as we age—those lovely round apple cheeks that make babies so pinchable are gradually absorbed. The solution to volume loss is not a face-lift, which pulls skin tight and taut over a bony skeleton, so skin can resemble a tambourine. And not a young tambourine at that. The solution is to fill up the envelope with a filler that mimics the volume of youth.

I just love fillers. The sheer versatility of the many different types of fillers currently available, with more awaiting FDA approval, makes fillers wonderful for nearly everyone. They're the most cost-effective treatment for volume loss in the long run, because when done properly, they guarantee results and can make you look terrific without surgical intervention. They can immediately shave about ten to fifteen years off your face, without surgical intervention and without altering the natural appearance of your face. You'll still look like *you*, only rounder.

The most basic cause for complaint from my patients about fillers is that they aren't permanent. Not surprisingly, this isn't a downside for many of those who've had less than stellar results with doctors, as they know that the filler will wear off eventually, usually within a year.

Some of my patients also worry that they'll droop or sag *more* after the filler wears off. I reassure them that this won't happen. For one thing, fillers wear off gradually, so it's not as if you go to bed one night looking rested and youthful, and wake up the next morning looking as if you'd just added twenty years to your skin. If anything, regular use of fillers means you'll sag *less*, because one of the benefits of fillers is that they may help stimulate your own collagen production, and this means more youthful-looking skin *after* the filler is gone. Also, because the lines have been filled in, they won't be getting deeper, as they might have been if left untreated. I believe that the more you use fillers, the greater the possibility of a buildup over time, so the less often you have to come back for more.

The question of which filler to use for volume loss is a subjective one, so be sure to discuss all the options carefully with your dermatologist. I find the synthetic fillers, such as Restylane, to be the easiest to control, with the most predictable results. Other dermatologists swear by fat injections.

Often, a mix of different substances gives optimal results. That's the real beauty of fillers—it's all about combining and tissue tailoring. And this is where the skill of your dermatologist is crucial. No matter which injectible substance is used, its success is entirely technique-dependent. The injections need to go where the *defect* (doctor lingo for wrinkle or line) is. If a wrinkle is superficial, the injection must be superficial, with a filler made with the tiniest particles. If the substance is too thick, it will cause bumps in the skin. Medium wrinkles need deeper injections, and so on. Be sure that your doctor is experienced with all the substances available, so you can have your treatment customized. I would be very suspicious of any physician who tells you that you need only one kind of filler to treat all the different types of wrinkles on your face. Always discuss the pros and cons prior to injection—and don't be afraid to ask questions.

Another question to discuss is when to stop. I've seen some big faces walking around that are truly frightening, because women keep asking doctors for more, more, more—and they're getting it. A judicious hand will help you look years better, no doubt about it. But you can't look twenty-five when you're fifty-five. You've got to be realistic about what fillers can and cannot do. They can't make a woman of a certain age, with a certain girth, look like Angelina Jolie or Natalie Portman. But they can make you look like a more youthful version of *you*.

What Can a Filler Do? Fillers are substances injected into the skin with a hypodermic needle to fill in lines and wrinkles. They replace lost volume in soft tissue, giving a lifting effect and restoring youthful contours to the face—in essence, giving you a "volume face-lift."

Injectibles can fill in superficial wrinkles, such as crow's-feet; moderate wrinkles and lines, such as the naso-labial folds, marionette lines, and cheek lines; and deep lines and furrows, such as the most pronounced naso-labial folds, marionette lines, and creases in the cheeks and elsewhere on the face. They can plump up thin lips and lift up the corners of a drooping mouth. They can fatten up thin earlobes, iron out earlobe creases, and plump up hands. They can round out a pointed chin and smooth the hollows under the eyes (what I call the "Restylane pillow," as it provides a pad around the eye and it makes you look rested). They can smooth out the jawline and lift and smooth the neck.

No topical cream will ever work as effectively as an injected filler.

What Can't a Filler Do? Fill large pores. Eliminate fat. Dynamic wrinkles, such as those on the forehead, are better treated with Botox.

Let's take a look at the many kinds of fillers.

COLLAGEN

Collagen is the grandmama of all fillers. It's been used in different medical procedures for over a century, so its efficacy has long been proven.

Collagen, as you know, is the protein component of skin. The collagen used for injection comes from two sources: bovine (from cow hooves and skin, called Zyderm 1, Zyderm 2, and Zyplast), or porcine (from pig tendons, called Evolence); and human (from infant foreskins, called CosmoDerm and Cosmo-Plast).

Zyderm was first approved by the FDA in 1981, and Zyplast in 1984. The difference between them is that Zyplast is cross-linked, so it will last longer, and Zyderm is not. The big problem with them is the unavoidable need to test for allergies to bovine collagen. This collagen is quite similar to human collagen, but at least 3 percent of the population remains allergic to it. It is mandatory to have a series of tests, done on the arm, spaced out over four weeks, to ensure you aren't one of the unlucky ones. Studies have shown that 1 out of 1,000 patients can, when double-tested (two skin tests), have a treatment-site reaction of redness and swelling. Although this is a temporary reaction, it means bovine collagen is off-limits.

Zyderm 1 and Zyderm 2 are best for the treatment of superficial wrinkles: shallow, horizontal forehead lines, shallow scars, and crow's-feet. Zyplast is thicker, making it better for deeper wrinkles, furrows, the naso-labial fold, and deep scars, and to fill in lips.

Because CosmoDerm and CosmoPlast are derived from a human cell source, there will not be the same problem with their allergenicity. You won't need an initial skin test and can be injected the same day as your initial consultation. CosmoDerm has the same effect as Zyderm, and CosmoPlast has the same effect as Zyplast. Despite its relatively short duration, I think CosmoDerm is probably the best product out there to treat fine lines and wrinkles.

How Often Should I Have Collagen? Zyplast and CosmoPlast last about three to six months. CosmoDerm and Zyderm last about three to four months.

Pain Factor All collagen syringes come premixed with a local anesthetic, lidocaine, which makes their injection about as pain-free as it comes. Still, I like to numb the skin with a topical anesthetic to ensure a painless procedure.

Recuperation Zyderm and Zyplast can cause redness and swelling, lasting for several days. CosmoDerm and CosmoPlast, on the other hand, can cause only mild redness, so they're great for instant gratification.

The other risk with collagen is that it can occlude a blood vessel at the injection site in the cheek or forehead. If this happens, the blood vessel supplying oxygen to the skin is now blocked, so the tissue above it dies. The result is a wound that might scar. Fortunately, this is a rare occurrence.

FAT TRANSFER

You'll never have to worry about allergic reactions to fat injections, as this fat will be harvested from your own body's cells.

Fat transfer is a two-part procedure. After a short liposuction procedure, where a small canula is inserted into the desired areas and fat is removed (usually from the abdomen, hips, or buttocks), it's then transferred to the face via injections. Some dermatologists do the extraction and inject small amounts over a period of time, usually about every three to four weeks for up to a year, until there is a complete correction. Others inject larger volumes at one time and try to do the correction all at once, which seems to last longer but has a longer recuperation time. Some dermatologists put the fat in a freezer to preserve it; others use only freshly harvested fat every time.

The big drawback to fat is that no one has yet been able to figure out how to make it stick. Some patients look incredible for a few months, or even a year or so, and then the replaced volume seems to disappear all at once. Others found that the fat didn't stick at all, making the procedure a (painful) loss.

For that reason—fat's variable duration, especially when you're injecting smaller amounts—the jury's still out on fat transfer. It's not my treatment of choice, although many of my colleagues swear by it. First, the liposuction procedure can hurt and is invasive—and expensive. The fat must be stored properly in freezers. Monthly injections are time-consuming. And the needles used to inject the fat are much larger than those used for other injectibles, so they hurt more.

On the other hand, there will always be a lifetime supply of fresh fat available, with no risk of any immune reaction. A technique where tiny droplets of fat are placed throughout the whole face, in particular building up areas of concavity, such as the temples, under and around the eyes, cheeks, the naso-labial fold, and in the lips, may give good results. But I still prefer collagen and Restylane. They last longer, they're more predictable, and you don't have to endure the extraction process. Many of my patients who've had both fat transfer and other injectibles swear they won't go through the fat transfer process again!

How Often Should I Have Fat Transfer? The results vary—anywhere from a few weeks to a few years. Sometimes there is still some slight improvement after a few years, but much diminished from the initial filling.

Pain Factor For large areas of liposuction, you're usually sedated, but for fat transfer, you'll only need a relatively small amount extracted, so the procedure will be done under local anesthesia. It still can hurt if a blood vessel is inadvertently nicked. The fat injections hurt more than other injectibles, as fat is much thicker than synthetics. Topical anesthetic cream is always used.

Recuperation Compression bandages at the harvesting site will need to be worn for up to a week, and the pain at the site can be pretty bad for a day or so, with soreness and limited mobility lasting up to a week or more.

There may be slight swelling and bruising at the injection sites. Once the needle is removed, there's no pain.

Fredric Brandt, MD

HYALURONIC ACIDS: RESTYLANE, HYLAFORM, AND JUVÉDERM

Hyaluronic acids are not really acids the way the AHAs are. They're polysaccharides, or natural sugars, that our bodies need in order to function properly. These sugars provide some of the skin's volume and pliability, filling in the space between the collagen and elastin fibers while delivering essential nutrients and hydration. If you imagine that your skin is a bowl of Jell-O, the gelatin would be the hyaluronic acids; strands of spaghetti floating in the Jell-O would be the collagen.

One of the most amazing properties of hyaluronic acid is that it can bind water up to a thousand times its volume in the skin. Its ability to hold on to water makes it an ideal ingredient in moisturizers. When injected, stabilized hyaluronic acid's ability to attract water helps keep its molecules plumped up. Hyaluronic acids are great to use because they're soft and pliable, like the collagen in your skin, so they actually *feel* like skin.

Hyaluronic acids are derived from either an animal source or a bacterial source. Unlike collagen, which comes from a bovine (cow) or porcine (pig) source, these substances do not normally trigger allergies, so no pre-treatment testing is needed. The animal-source hyaluronic acids are Hylaform and Hylaform Plus, derived from rooster combs. The non-animal stabilized hyaluronic acids, or NASHA, which I prefer to use, are derived from the by-products of the fermentation of strep bacteria—so you can rest assured that you are *not* being injected with the bacteria itself! This group includes the Restylane family (made by Medicis) and the Juvéderm family (made by Allergan). During the production process, acid is stabilized and cross-linked, which allows it to hold up better in the face. If not cross-linked, the product would dissipate completely within several hours of being injected. Basically, that explains the difference between the different brands; the NASHA is the same, but the stabilization process is slightly altered.

When the hyaluronic gel is filtered, as with the Restylane family of fillers, the size of its spherical particles changes. Larger filters and particles create Perlane; medium filters and particles create Restylane; and the smallest filters and particles create Restylane Fine Lines. Obviously, the larger the substance, the larger the needle. Perlane is used for deep wrinkles; Restylane for medium; and Restylane Fine Lines for the topmost, superficial lines and wrinkles. Since Restylane falls in the middle, it's great for replacing volume defects of mid to deeper lines. It can be used for facial contouring and to fill in around the eyes—basically anywhere on the face. And it's a great product for a lip enhancement.

The Restylane family includes, in ascending order of molecule size: Restylane Vital, with the smallest particle size, to improve skin elasticity and tone; Restylane Fine Lines Touch, for fine lines; Restylane; Restylane Lipp, tissue-tailored to be more viscous to work more effectively on the lips' natural anatomy; Perlane; and Restylane Sub-Q, which is also more viscous and designed to go deeper, to correct the deepest folds and wrinkles. Restylane Sub-Q will have more of a lifting effect when compared to other fillers, so it might be good for those considering surgery. Of these, only Restylane is approved by the FDA, but the others await imminent approval.

One of the best things about Restylane or other hyaluronic acids is that they can be dissolved. If you get a bump, or if your dermatologist was a bit heavy-handed, a substance called hyaluronidace breaks down what was injected. It's nice to know there's a safety valve with this particular injected substance.

In the fall of 2006, the FDA approved the Juvéderm family of hyaluronic acid fillers. Juvéderm has been used successfully in many other countries. Patients who've had it feel it may be a little smoother when it's injected, as there are no tiny particle beads in the gel. Instead, it comes in different viscosities to treat different types of wrinkles, so treatment can be fine-tuned. Because it's a smooth gel, this can reduce the possibility of an inflammatory reaction (such as swelling). Juvéderm 18 is used for fine lines; Juvéderm Ultra is best for medium wrinkles; and Juvéderm Ultraplus is the most dense and cross-linked, and is best for deep wrinkles and folds.

Captique, from Inamed, is another filler that I'm not crazy about, as it doesn't last as long as Restylane—only about two to three months. It's also a non-animal stabilized form of hyaluronic acid.

How Often Should I Have Restylane? Restylane usually lasts for about six months. Some of my repeat patients report that it lasts up to a year in the cheek area. The more you're treated, the longer the Restylane lasts.

Fredric Brandt, MD

Pain Factor The needles used are ultra-fine. The skin is numbed before treatment with topical anesthetic, so most patients have minimal pain.

Recuperation It depends on the amount injected. If a large area, such as the cheeks and the jowls, has been treated, bruising can persist for up to two weeks.

Unlike collagen, theoretically you can't be allergic to hyaluronic acid. There are, however, trace amounts of protein in the product—remnants from the bacterial fermentation or animal processing, so there are very rare cases of temporary allergic reaction to those substances.

POLYLACTIC ACID

Polylactic acid is a substance that, once injected, is metabolized by the body into lactose and eventually broken down. Called Sculptra, it's been approved in the United States for compassionate use in HIV patients who suffer from *lipoatrophy*, or a severe loss of fat in their faces that gives them a cadaverous appearance.

Sculptra is used off-label for facial augmentation and volume replacement, and to fill deep lines. It's not meant to be used on fine lines, and never in the lips, but it's great for adding volume to the face and giving what I call my "filler face-lift."

As Sculptra is injected deep in the skin, it has to be done extremely carefully, in very, very small amounts. Be sure your dermatologist is experienced with its use.

How Often Should I Have Sculptra? The initial treatment is once a month for three to five treatments. Sculptra lasts about two years.

Pain Factor The skin is numbed with topical anesthetic, so the procedure should have minimal pain.

Recuperation As with Restylane, there may be redness, swelling, and/or bruising.

There have been reports that some patients have developed little nodules in the skin, small lumps that are palpable—and visible. Needless to say, this

92

could be a distressing side effect. The obvious question is whether this is due to poor injection technique (injected too superficially) or to problems with the product. My guess is it's probably a combination of both. None of my patients have had any problems with Sculptra.

SYNTHETIC FILLERS: SILICONE AND ARTEFILL

Some of my patients only want a permanent filler. Actually, they don't just want it. They *demand* it. I do explain to them that no filler is truly "permanent," because new wrinkles will always continue to form and skin will always continue its gravity-led descent down where you don't want it to go!

Always think very carefully and discuss any questions or worries with your dermatologist if you're considering any permanent fillers. The bottom line about them is that they can be recommended for specific situations, as long as you are aware of the risks and the history of previous problems with these permanent fillers.

Be certain that whomever you choose to inject you has had years of experience working with these substances. With any permanent injectible or implants, there can be several kinds of problems. They can be material-innate or injector-innate, or both. Material-innate problems are due to the material itself. Injector-innate or technique problems are bumps and lumps due to bad injection technique. If the substance is temporary, the bad results will eventually go away (or, with Restylane, they can be erased immediately. With a permanent product, they won't. Some kind of intervention is warranted, and it might not be pretty!

SILICONE

Silicone, the best-known and the most unfairly judged of all the synthetic fillers, was used for years in the 1960s through the 1980s. Many of my patients of a certain age have had silicone injections decades ago—and have completely forgotten about it until I ask them. Most of them certainly look much better now than they would if they hadn't had the initial silicone injections. Needless to say, if they've had any problems, they would have remembered that!

Silicone, now called Silikon 1000, is a purified inorganic compound, ap-

93

Fredric Brandt, MD

proved by the FDA for ophthalmic use and dispensed by dermatologists off-label. It works in the same manner that an oyster creates a pearl when an irritant becomes trapped inside its shell. When silicone is injected, your body forms collagen as a protective wall around this foreign substance.

There are several cautions with silicone:

Problems arose in the past when doctors used impure, not medical grade, silicone, which triggered reactions.

You must be absolutely assured that your dermatologist knows exactly what he or she is doing. Silicone needs a deft hand and a specific technique. It should only be injected one micro-droplet at a time, no more than 0.05 cc. You may end up with a hundred little pricks, with a total of no more than 0.8 total cc's.

Unfortunately, there are some physicians or other practitioners who don't know how to inject silicone. They either inject too much in one place, or too much overall, which can cause lumps in the skin called granulomas. I once treated a patient who was an otherwise sane woman who'd gone to see some shady character who worked out of a hotel room, and she'd had a horrible reaction. Luckily, she responded to the cortisone I used to bring down the swelling, but it took years before she finally looked like herself again. Another patient had seen an overzealous cosmetic surgeon who inflated her lips to gigantic proportions, and they were hard and lumpy, like marbles.

Years ago, when those who were allergic to collagen were having reactions because allergenicity testing wasn't yet the recommended protocol, there were cases where doctors felt they had to resort to cutting out the damaged area completely, leaving a visible scar (which was, of course, far worse than the original defect). Now I can usually treat adverse reactions to silicone, which are still fairly rare with other injectibles, so surgery isn't necessary. For those who do develop granulomas, even when only a minute amount of silicone has been injected, don't panic and demand that they be cut out. Cortisone may be able to treat them and shrink them down.

Silicone has a reputation as a substance that migrates to other parts of the body. Certainly the controversy over silicone breast implants has fueled that debate, although the sheer volume of a breast implant is vastly greater than what should be injected into a face. Again, from my years of experience handing silicone, I'd say that this reputation might be overstated. I believe that the problem isn't so much that the silicone shifts, but that as the face ages and shifts, the placement of the silicone shifts too. Remember that even "permanent" fillers change over time, because you are still going through the aging process and things, well, move around (and usually not where you want them to go).

If silicone has appeared to shift due to inevitable sags and wrinkles, or if it wears away to the point where the original injection site is visible, such as in a scar, the simple solution is to add a little bit more silicone and correct around it.

Trust me when I say that jowls are going to develop whether you have silicone or not. It's certainly not the silicone that's responsible for jowls!

What Can Silicone Do? Fill in scars, defects, cleft lips, thin lips, deeper lines, and moderate wrinkles. Add volume to the cheek area.

What Can't Silicone Do? Give immediate gratification!

How Often Should I Get Silicone? Silicone must be a very slow process. The injections of the micro-droplets should be spaced at least a month apart. It can take anywhere from six months to a year to see the ultimate results. After that, silicone is relatively permanent.

Pain Factor The skin is numbed before treatment with topical anesthetic, so pain should be minimal.

Recuperation There might be occasional bruising.

ARTEFILL

ArteFill, which was previously called Arteplast, then Artecoll, is the first permanent injectible filler to be approved by the FDA for the treatment of wrinkles. It's a combination of 80 percent by volume bovine collagen, which serves as carrier material for the remaining 20 percent of synthetic Plexiglas-type particle microspheres (polymethylmethacrylate, or PMMA), about 30 to 42 microns in diameter. There are more than 6 million microspheres per cc. When this substance is injected deep into the skin, the collagen carrier is gradually absorbed into the body over about one to three months, and the microspheres remain permanently. As with silicone, new collagen is formed around them—your own collagen encapsulates the microspheres, producing and maintaining a filler effect.

ArteFill has had a checkered evolution over the years. There were reports that the earlier versions triggered inflammatory reactions to the microspheres as a few years went by. Swelling began to appear and granulomas were forming, visible enough to see and disturbingly hard to the touch. This was especially disturbing for anyone who'd had their lips injected. The problem seemed to have been with the purity of the microspheres. (The collagen portion requires prior testing and has not been an issue with this filler.) As Arteplast and Artecoll were permanent, the fixes for these lumps were either steroid injections or surgery that left a visible scar.

According to the manufacturer, Artes Medical, ArteFill has fixed that problem. The microspheres are more uniform, less fragmented, and have been purified, so the inflammatory reactions shouldn't occur.

What Can ArteFill Do? Treat deep lines and moderate wrinkles, scars, even on the nose, and fill thin lips or earlobes.

What Can't ArteFill Do? Treat superficial or fine lines.

How Often Should I Get ArteFill? It may take a few treatments, spaced at least one month apart, for the final effect. Once done, the results are permanent.

Pain Factor Each syringe is pre-loaded with lidocaine, so there should be minimal pain. It's best to have a topical anesthetic cream, just to be sure pain from the needle penetration is minimized.

Recuperation There may be a bit of temporary swelling, redness, or tenderness.

BONY SUBSTANCE

Radiesse is calcium hydroxyl apetite (Catla), a synthetic bony-type substance. It's approved for laryngeal injections and is used off-label as a soft-tissue filler.

Since the NASHA fillers and collagen are more physiologically compatible with the skin, I don't use Radiesse. I don't think it lasts significantly longer than Restylane, which would outweigh some of the side effects. With improper technique, lumps and bumps can form in the skin.

COMING ATTRACTIONS

As technology improves, many new injectibles are being created and refined. The FDA is quite stringent on its rules for approval, needing years of double-blind testing (where neither the physician nor the patients know what's in the syringe) before receiving approval. Many injectible fillers available in Europe and South America have been used safely there for years, but are still deep in the FDA pipeline.

Some of the most promising new injectibles are:

- Evolence. This is a pig-derived collagen that's supposed to last for a year or two, without the allergenicity of bovine collagen.

- Isolagen. This is a revolutionary process where a tiny piece of skin, the size of an eraser head, is removed from the back of a patient's ear and sent to a certified lab. There the fibroblast cells within the collagen are grown in a laboratory setting. Next, they're returned to the physician, who has a short window of opportunity to inject the new fibroblasts back into the skin. Ideally, your skin will use these fibroblasts to spur the production of entirely new collagen. It usually takes about four months for any results to appear. In addition, cryogenic storage of cultured cells may also permit patients to receive future treatments with cells that were harvested when the patient was younger.

  Isolagen is approved for use in the United Kingdom, where it has successfully treated lines and wrinkles, as well as burn scars and acne scars. It may do more than just work as a filler, because I've seen reports and pictures of burn victims and patients with scarring from laser resurfacing, and it seemed to resurface the skin as well. Live cell therapy definitely has potential, but until I can test Isolagen myself, I must reserve judgment. My Dermatology Research Institute will be conducting clinical trials for Isolagen during 2007, and I'm a principal investigator in this FDA trial.

- Profill. This is a double-cross-linked hyaluronic acid. It has a different cross-linking process, and each syringe has lidocaine in it, so the injections should be a little less painful.

- Recombinant collagen. This is collagen that will be entirely lab created—made from genetically engineered DNA. This is still in the laboratory stage.

ARE PERMANENT IMPLANTS SAFE?

Implants are permanent substances inserted under the skin in a surgical procedure. They can be derived from biologic materials, such as cadaver skin (called AlloDerm), or from synthetic materials, such as Gore-Tex.

Implants were more popular years ago, especially for the lips and nasolabial fold, when the only alternative was collagen. Fillers have improved so radically in the last few years that I don't recommend any permanent implants for the face. I've found the implants to be very unpredictable. They can shrink over time, and they can protrude over the skin. And as they're permanent, if there are problems, or if you don't like them, the only way to fix them is with surgery, which can leave a scar and brings its attendant risks.

With cadaver skin, there's always the worry about its origin, and how well it was screened for disease transmission or viruses. A recent scandal where body parts were illegally and improperly removed from diseased corpses and implanted in thousands of people (usually for non-cosmetic reasons) has cast a terrifying light on the market for human tissue.

I think it's much wiser to stick to the temporary fillers from reputable manufacturers. If you don't like the results, you won't have to live with them forever.

98

WHAT IF I'M NEEDLE-PHOBIC?

When I use fillers, I might be making dozens of tiny injections over the course of the procedure. I use very strong topical anesthetic creams to numb the skin, which takes anywhere from thirty to forty-five minutes. I sometimes use nerve blocks to numb the lips and cheek area. These are Xylocaine shots in the gums, similar to what you might get at the dentist. Most patients are familiar with those kinds of shots so there's next to no anxiety about them.

Still, I've had patients who've gotten nearly 100 injections in their face without a whimper, yet when it comes time to draw their blood, they're extremely upset and ready to faint. Eyes wide shut is the only solution to blood draws!

Some of my patients are also more sensitive to pain than others, and I help them with relaxation breathing techniques. When I do use injectibles on my patients, I do one side at a time, then show them the results. It usually wows them in an amazing way—and helps in case there is any discomfort, since they're so pleased with the results that pain magically vanishes!

Don't hesitate to speak up if you have anxiety prior to any treatment.

Muscle Freezers

I don't think it's an understatement to claim that Botox and its new cousin, Reloxin (which used to be called Dysport), have revolutionized the treatment of aging skin. I've been a fan of Botox since it came onto the market, for it is unsurpassed in its versatility. Not only can it remove lines and wrinkles in certain areas of the face, but it allows you to treat large areas with dramatic results—and no surgery.

That is, when the syringe is wielded by the right hands, of course. In the wrong hands, Botox can be a disaster! You need only look at the preternaturally frozen faces of Hollywood superstars, whose foreheads are as strangely smooth and immobile as a polished marble statue of Aphrodite, to see the results of Botox gone bad.

There are seven types of the botulinum toxin, ranging from A to G. The

Fredric Brandt, MD

Botox commonly used to treat wrinkles and other skin concerns is a type A toxin, a highly purified protein produced by the *Clostridium botulinum* bacterium. Botox and Reloxin work by temporarily blocking the nerve impulses that control muscle movement. This restricts your ability to contract your facial muscles. No movement of the muscles underneath the skin means no wrinkles on the skin above them.

The FDA first approved Botox in December 1989 for the treatment of eye muscle disorders, and again in December 2000 for cervical dystonia, a neurological disorder that causes severe neck and shoulder contractions. In the meantime, physicians impressed with what it could do were using it "off-label," meaning for other than the specific FDA-designated intent (which is perfectly medically acceptable), when they realized that one of the unforeseen side effects of Botox's medical use was the smoothing of wrinkles. After years of testing, the FDA finally approved Botox Cosmetic product for glabellar lines (between the eyebrows) in April 2002. Reloxin is expected to be approved in 2008.

Botox and Reloxin are both type A toxins, but they have different qualities of proteins and carriers due to different manufacturing processes. Reloxin will probably have some slightly different characteristics than Botox. Some of the testing results have shown that it may diffuse more, meaning that it might affect a slightly wider area. That may be great when you want to treat a large area, such as the neck, but may not be great when you want more of a localized effect, such as for frown lines.

Another FDA-approved toxin, Myobloc, is a botulinum toxin type B. When it was first approved, hopes for it were high, as it took effect more quickly than Botox, usually within a day. But it lasts for only about two months, so that even pushing it to higher doses made it too expensive for regular use. It is rarely used anymore.

When I first began using Botox more than ten years ago, patients were palpably anxious about the fact that I was injecting them with a toxin that is lethal in large doses. There's really nothing to worry about. A lethal dose of Botox for humans is approximately 3,000 units. A standard Botox injection for glabellar, or frown lines ranges from 25 up to about 75 units. It's a dosage level that can never be remotely toxic.

Botox has become so popular, and such a buzzword, that I often have young patients (late teens and twenties) who ask for it without really understanding what Botox can or cannot do. Normally, I don't recommend it for people under the age of about twenty-five or so, but every patient is different. Particularly in Miami, where so many of my patients have been worshiping the sun since they were children, I see a tremendous amount of sun damage and premature wrinkling. That kind of patient might be a better candidate for Botox at twenty-six than the average person in New York who wears sunscreen every day. I do spend a lot of time dissuading new patients that Botox is not a cure-all for sun worship. Often, all they need is a lesson in how to best protect themselves from the sun along with, perhaps, a light peel.

One of the other problems with Botox's popularity is that anyone with a medical license can inject it. But the product itself is only a small part of the process. A specific kind of spatial skill is a prerequisite for anyone claiming to know how to use Botox. It's like an artist's work—the paint and the brush might be identical, but fifty different artists will create fifty different styles of paintings. So you can't judge Botox by some of the results you can peruse on the bad plastic surgery websites.

If too much Botox is injected, you can wind up looking like Mr. Softy, weirdly soft and smooth. Too much Botox can also cause the brows to drop, as the surrounding muscles can't pull them up (temporarily, of course).

If too little Botox is injected, you'll just be wasting your money. With Botox, you really do get what you pay for. Cut-rate injectors are watering down the original solution, so you may have a good initial response, but it will wear off quite quickly.

I think it's beyond crazy to allow anyone without a license to inject Botox into your face, or anywhere else. I've treated the aftereffects of patients who thought they could save a little money by going to Botox parties where alleged experts were sticking anyone in sight. Treat your body with respect, and only allow a physician with years of experience handling injectibles to touch your skin!

What Can Botox and Reloxin Do? Muscle freezers are unparalleled for the treatment of forehead lines. When skillfully injected, they will have the same effect as a brow lift.

They're great for eliminating lines around the eyes, and the under-eye bulge, to open the eyes up.

Around the mouth, they can treat the vertical lines, caused by the pursing movement of smoking, above and below the lips. They can also treat the "marionette" lines running from the outside corner of the mouth to the chin.

They can literally lift up the tip of the nose.

On the chin, they can remove dimpling and remove some mild to moderate jowling. They can lift the jawline.

On the neck, they can lift the skin, treating the lines and bands of the neck, eliminating the prominent *platysmal bands* (the muscle that runs from the chin to the neck).

Botox can also be a terrific adjunct to cosmetic surgery. It can be used after a face-lift, especially when patients have a lot of tension after their skin has been pulled back. When you relax the muscles with Botox, there's less tension on the skin and better, more natural results. Or, with a forehead lift, Botox can correct symmetries and asymmetries.

Botox does have a slight cumulative effect. The more you get, the longer I believe it lasts. Let's say you had an unconscious tendency to wrinkle your brow when you concentrate, as many do. If the muscles involved in allowing that wrinkle to happen aren't being used, even when you try to frown, nothing will happen. You may lose the habit entirely, in which case the wrinkles will not reform. Wrinkles caused by squinting, however, will come back.

Botox has also been used to treat lines on the chest and migraine headaches, and to eliminate excessive sweating under the arms and on the palms (called *hyperhidrosis*), as well as tackle certain symptoms of Parkinson's disease and Bell's palsy.

What Can't Botox and Reloxin Do? Work right away. They take a few days for the full effect to kick in.

Nor can they last longer than three to six months. Botox and Reloxin are not permanent, so they gradually wear off. As they block the nerves that "talk" to the muscle, eventually your own cells figure out how to bypass them. This irreversible chemical reaction can be a relief if your doctor was overzealous and parts of you look bizarrely unlined while the rest is sagging.

Botox and Reloxin are not fillers. They can't be used to enlarge lips. They can't replace lost volume, so they can't fill in a large area such as a cheek. (Only a filler will work.) They can't treat sagging in the cheeks or the naso-labial fold.

Remember that the deeper your line is, the deeper the wrinkle at rest. If you have furrows that your dermatologist believes will respond eventually to Botox, don't have unrealistic expectations. It might take several sessions over the course of a year for the wrinkle to diminish.

How Often Can I Have Botox or Reloxin Injections? Typically, patients come in every three to four months.

Pain Factor The skin can be numbed with a topical anesthetic cream first. Many patients report that they feel no pain and are bothered (if they're bothered at all) by the slightly crunchy sound of the material being injected. The needles are very fine, about the size of acupuncture needles. The injections should be very quick, but if you're having a large area treated, it could take some time to do it. Most of my patients are not bothered at all and feel next to no discomfort.

Recuperation Time I tell my patients to use the muscles—frown, smile, talk animatedly—for two hours after treatment. The most common side effects are a headache or a strong feeling of heaviness. Rarely, there can be a temporary eyelid droop or nausea.

WHAT ABOUT GROWTH HORMONES?

Growth hormones are a new human experiment. A controlled study by Dr. Daniel Rudman showed that prescription injected synthetic human growth hormone increased muscle mass and decreased body fat in adult males. The study participants also reported better sleep, increased energy, and better muscle and skin tone. Because this study was done on a small population of elderly men, I don't feel we can extrapolate it to be a panacea for aging.

The only proven way for them to work is to inject these hormones daily or several times a week. While this may have beneficial effects, the hormones may also increase your risk for diabetes, arthritis, congestive heart failure, or cancer. There have not been enough long-term, controlled studies to see if the benefits are sustainable or if they outweigh the risk of injecting these hormones.

There are liquid, spray, and pill forms that reportedly give the benefit of human growth hormones, but there are no studies that show these forms are of any benefit.

If you want to risk your life and your health in order to take hormones that have not been tested over the long haul, and therefore may be extremely risky, it's certainly your prerogative. We haven't yet discovered a magic potion to stop the aging process. Try cutting sugar out of your diet, and follow a good exercise regime and a healthy lifestyle; you will feel better, lose weight, and avoid being responsible for creating your own demise.

Chemical Peels

Chemical peels speed up skin cell turnover, making them skin resurfacing and exfoliation treatments. They're usually done with some form of an acidic compound (usually AHAs), either glycolic or salicylic acid, gluconolactone, resorcinol, trichloroacetic (TCA), phenol, or a combination of several of them. A Jessner's solution peel combines resorcinol, salicylic acid, and the anti-oxidant lactic acid. A dermatologist-supervised peel is much stronger than an OTC peel. An OTC might contain 10 percent to 20 percent glycolic acid, for instance, and a deep phenol peel can go up to 70 percent. A beta-hydroxy acid in the form of salicylic acid usually has a concentration of 20 percent to 30 percent (OTC salicylic acid peels are usually about 2 percent).

Peels can be tricky, however, especially the stronger ones tackling medium and deep layers of skin. If done improperly, and with a skewed pH balance, post-inflammatory hyperpigmentation (uneven skin tone, spots, blotches) can result, especially in those with darker skin tones.

Deep peels done with phenol have pretty much been replaced by non-ablative, or peeling, lasers, which don't burn the skin the way acids do and have more predictable results and a shorter downtime. Bear in mind that deep peels are serious business. They do go down deep, but the result is a severe response, with raw, wounded, oozing skin for two to three weeks, and pinkness for several months. There's also a risk of scarring, as well as hypopigmentation, where the new skin is lighter than the surrounding skin of the untreated neck and body.

Bottom line with deep peels: You must trust that your dermatologist knows what he or she is doing, because the burning can be severe and damage can be permanent if a strict protocol is not followed. As with everything in cosmetic dermatology, technique is crucial. There are many variables when doing a peel—the pH (acid balance) of the peeling solution, skin type, coloring, skin thickness, prepping the skin, acid concentration, and more. Luckily, I don't see too much of those kinds of severe burns anymore, as the deepest peel, done with phenol, has pretty much been replaced by the different lasers that have less variables to worry about.

What Can Peels Do? By removing the dead layer of cells (stratum corneum) on the topmost layer of skin, exfoliating peels erase very fine, superficial lines, hyperpigmentation spots, and smooth uneven or coarse texture. Pores become unclogged, skin is softer, and acne is improved. Peels are rated according to their strength of the peel: very superficial, superficial, medium, and deep. The stronger the peel, obviously, the more profound the effect.

Very superficial and superficial peels can definitely give your skin a certain glow and radiance. They can also even out hyperpigmentation.

Medium peels are quite effective for those with fine wrinkling and hyperpigmentation.

Deep peels are used for those with severe sun damage, with many crosshatched lines and skin with a rough, leathery texture. They will stimulate collagen regeneration, with visible results. They can also provide a slight tightening effect.

What Can't Peels Do? Replace lost volume. Very superficial and superficial peels can only treat surface fine lines and wrinkles.

How Often Should I Have a Peel? Peels usually need to be done in a series for the best results.

For superficial peels, I usually recommend a series of four, spaced about three to four weeks apart, for optimal results. This can be repeated every year to keep skin in optimum condition.

Medium peels need to be repeated no more than once a year, if that.

For deep peels you should need to suffer through the pain and raw skin only once or twice in your lifetime.

Pain Factor Very superficial and superficial peels shouldn't hurt. There might be a little tingling.

Medium peels feel like tingling or burning during the procedure. There should be no pain once you're home.

Deep peels hurt. A lot. Sedation is mandatory during the procedure, so it will be painless. Once the sedation wears off, prescription painkillers will be needed.

Recuperation Very superficial and superficial peels have little downtime, if any. There might be some peeling, which can be covered up by moisturizing creams.

Medium peels necessitate a recovery period of about one week. The skin turns red, then brown, then flakes off. After ten days, you should be completely back to normal.

Deep peels trigger such an extreme response to the skin that you will not want to see anyone (or be seen) for two weeks. Makeup can be applied only after at least two weeks. And then your skin will stay red to pink for several long months. A strict maintenance regimen must be followed or you can scar or get an even worse burn.

Lasers

Lasers have exploded in popularity over the last few years, and almost everybody with aging concerns can benefit from them. Lasers are amazing skin resurfacers. They've pretty much replaced the harder-to-control acid peels, and they can work incredibly well for those who have deeper, more problematic cheek wrinkles that don't respond to retinoid creams or other procedures.

If you're considering any kind of laser treatment, be an educated consumer, choose your laser carefully according to your skin coloration and specific needs, and see a trained dermatologist in a physician-supervised facility. You want a doctor wielding the device. (Some physicians lease the lasers during a specific time period, such as one day a week, to do all the procedures; if so, this should be explained to you prior to treatment. You need to be sure that the physician is extremely familiar with the laser you're considering as well as its technical status.)

Lasers aren't toys. Signing on for one is a serious commitment. It can hurt. It can be expensive. There can be downtime. In untrained hands, lasers can wreak havoc. But when done properly, they can have a remarkable effect on your appearance — literally resurfacing your skin.

Laser stands for Light Amplification by the Stimulation of Emission of Radiation. A laser is a concentrated, intense wavelength of light that's attracted to different things in your skin. So depending on what you want to accomplish, the physician will choose a wavelength of light that's attracted to a specific target. If you want to tackle your hyperpigmentation spots, you'd choose a laser that's attracted to melanin, the pigment in your skin. If you have rosacea, you'd choose a vascular laser that's attracted to red spots and blood vessels. For wrinkles, you'd choose a laser attracted to the water in the skin, which absorbs the light. When that happens, wrinkles, sun damage, and hyperpigmentation are absorbed and disappear.

What Can Lasers Do? Treat and minimize wrinkles and lines. Not only do they exfoliate the skin's surface, but they also increase collagen production as well as tighten collagen fibers, making skin more pliable and improving its texture. Some can perform toning and tightening, especially of the pores. They can also remove hyperpigmentation (brown spots), scars, stretch marks, broken blood vessels, hair, and tattoos. The higher the wavelength of the laser, the deeper it penetrates into the skin. The lower, the more superficial.

What Can't Lasers Do? Non-ablative lasers can't "lift" skin the way surgery can, although some of the lasers have a tightening and lifting effect. No laser can replace lost volume.

There are several kinds of lasers: non-ablative (non-burning), ablative, pigment and vascular, and hybrid.

Fredric Brandt, MD

NON-ABLATIVE LASERS

Ablative means removing the surface of the skin. Non-ablative lasers don't remove or peel the surface of the skin, which is why there's no burning or downtime—there's literally no wounding. You can have a treatment on your lunch hour, then go back to work and no one will have a clue! They aren't necessarily more effective than ablative lasers, but they are safer; they all have cooling devices that cool the surface of the skin so the energy can be delivered deeper into the skin without causing a burn.

The most popular non-ablative lasers are the CoolTouch, Smoothbeam, NLite (photorejuvenation), and Gemini (formerly the Aura and Lyra, now combined).

How Often Should I Have a Non-Ablative Laser Treatment? Because these treatments are gentle, a series of four to six is necessary before seeing any results. This series can be repeated as needed. Some of my patients love non-ablative lasers so much that they come nearly every month.

Pain Factor None to minimal.

Recuperation None.

ABLATIVE LASERS

When the carbon dioxide (CO_2) laser first came out, dermatologists were thrilled, because we finally had a new weapon—other than phenol peels or dermabrasion—to treat deep wrinkles and years of sun damage.

The CO_2 laser is heavy artillery, the most powerful laser there is for treating deep lines. It's also recommenced for anyone with fair skin and crepey wrinkles, especially on the cheeks and around the lips. No other procedure works as effectively at shrinking this kind of fine, diffuse wrinkling, or at tackling deeper, more entrenched wrinkles.

Not surprisingly, any procedure that works as deeply into the skin as a CO_2 laser has attendant risks, equivalent to those of a deep phenol peel. The

108

skin has been injured. There may be hypopigmentation, scarring, or infections. Sedation is necessary, and healing is tough.

How Often Should I Have a CO_2 Laser? Once or twice in your lifetime is more than enough.

Pain Factor The procedure itself is painful, so you should be prescribed an oral prescription painkiller. Pain will be mild to moderate post-procedure. Then it will lessen to the feeling of a severe sunburn, with attendant irritation.

Recuperation Expect up to two weeks of raw, oozing, crusting skin. You will not want to leave the house. Redness will persist for several months.

    The Erbium:YAG (Er:YAG) laser is also successful at treating moderate wrinkles and sun damage. Its effects are equivalent to that of a moderate peel. It causes less damage to surrounding tissue, so it has fewer side effects and less recuperation time.

How Often Should I Have an Erbium:YAG Laser? It depends on the depth. A light one can be done once a year, a moderate to deep treatment once every five years.

Pain Factor Mild to moderate.

Recuperation Skin will be sore and red for a week. It will remain red for about a month.

PIGMENT LASERS

These lasers target the brown spots of hyperpigmentation, usually caused by excessive production of melanin, triggered by sun exposure.

    These lasers are called Q-switched ruby, Q-switched alexandrite, Q-switched Nd:YAG, and Aura. They use tiny pulses of concentrated energy to remove hyperpigmentation spots on the face, hands, shoulders, and chest.

Fredric Brandt, MD

How Often Can I Have a Pigment Laser Treatment? As often as necessary to treat hyperpigmentation spots and freckles on the face. (If you keep going out in the sun, though, new hyperpigmentation spots will form and the procedure will have to be repeated.)

Pain Factor Topical anesthesia is used, so pain should be minimal.

Recuperation The skin will redden and scabs will form, for a week or two. You can wear makeup after a week. The hands, arms, and legs take much longer to heal; the further down from the face, the longer the healing process. Redness can persist on the face for more than a month and on the body for several months.

VASCULAR LASERS

Like the pigment lasers, vascular lasers target specific colors—in this case, they go after the red spectrum by targeting hemoglobin, the pigment that turns blood its typical red color, within blood vessels.

These lasers are the VersaPulse, Aura, and Vbeam. They treat redness, rosacea, and birthmarks on the face caused by broken or dilated blood vessels.

How Often Should I Have a Vascular Laser Treatment? As needed, depending on your specific condition.

Pain Factor Little to none.

Recuperation Next to none.

HYBRID LASERS (FRAXEL)

Fraxel (short for "fractional") is a laser that produces thousands of tiny but deep columns of treatment in your skin, called microthermal treatment zones. As it selectively heats certain microns of skin, like a grid, there's less wounding of the skin.

Fraxel can improve skin texture, wrinkles, and hyperpigmentation. I'm not yet convinced that Fraxel works as well on deep lines and wrinkles.

How Often Can I Have Fraxel? You'll need at least three to five sessions, spaced 3–5 weeks apart. It can be repeated every few years, as needed (more often if you don't protect your skin from the sun).

Pain Factor Fraxel is not as painful as a CO_2 laser, but pain is still mild to moderate. Oral prescription medication and topical anesthetic cream are used.

Recuperation There's slightly more downtime than with the non-ablative lasers, and there will be redness, swelling, and flaking post-treatment. Skin will appear to be bronzed for about three days.

WHEN THE NEEDLE'S NOT ENOUGH: WHEN IS COSMETIC SURGERY THE BEST OPTION?

One of my patients, Mrs. Twombley, came in a few weeks ago. She's had a lot of surgery and, in my opinion, she's been pulled way too much. I was busy injecting her, and she said, "I'm thinking of going to a plastic surgeon."

My hand holding the needle froze in midair. I looked at her in disbelief.

"I'll send you to Bellevue before I send you to a plastic surgeon!" I told Mrs. Twombley. "There's nothing left to pull!"

I've seen far too many patients like Mrs. Twombley. These women didn't have to endure numerous surgical procedures, ending up pulled and stretched to the limit. You'd think they'd look much younger, or much better, but they don't. They look *done*.

So they come to me in despair. They were told a face-lift would make them look perfect—and it didn't. Unfortunately, it's often when their real problems begin.

A face-lift isn't going to make you look perfect or eradicate all signs of aging. It's going to make you look tight. After a face-lift, your jawline will definitely be tighter.

What's the sense of looking pulled if you still look your age?

My goal isn't to make you look like you've had obvious work done. My goal is to make you look younger. That often isn't done with a scalpel. It's done with fillers. As you know by now, what ages you the most (aside from sun damage) is a loss of volume. Fillers replace that lost volume. A face-lift takes it away.

That said, sometimes cosmetic surgeons can do wonders with certain areas of the face and body. They can make tremendous improvements in your appearance. And one positive aspect of the television shows dealing with cosmetic surgery and the media coverage is to remove the stigma and secrecy that had once been attached to any elective procedure, especially face-lifts. The better informed you are, the more available the procedures, the more subtle the results, the easier it will be for you to find a qualified surgeon who believes, as I do, that less is often more.

That said, it's as easy to find a surgeon who likes to cut and doesn't know when to stop as it is to find a dermatologist who overinflates cheeks and lips with too much filler. I know how simple it is because I'm often treating the patients who are desperate for corrections. Sometimes I can help them. Sometimes I can't.

I also can't help the patients who are addicted to surgical procedures, and there are plenty of them. In my opinion, what they might need is professional counseling to help them understand their ambivalence and fears about their appearance (termed *body dysmorphic disorder*) rather than another operation.

My philosophy is that the goal of having your skin treated is to end up looking natural. You want to look like yourself. You don't want to look too tight. You don't want to look unnaturally smooth. You don't want to look freakish, with tip-tilted eyes that have been pulled at the corners, or with lips the size of your fingers, or with a forehead yanked so high your eyebrows are fixed in a position of permanent questioning. Most of all, you don't want to look *embalmed*.

Here's where I believe cosmetic surgery can be useful:

- Sagging upper eyelids. Excess skin in the eyelids can't be treated by a dermatologist.

- Fat accumulation under the eye. Some people have pooching-out bags under their eyes caused by excess fat deposits. This isn't the same situation as dark circles or hollows. Large pockets of fat under the eyes need to be surgically removed, but with a subtle hand. If too much fat is taken out, the area will appear hollow and need fillers in order to look normal.

- Bumps in the nose, or nose reduction. Botox in the tip of the nose can stop it from drooping, but no procedure at the dermatologist can rival a rhinoplasty for changing the shape of a nose.

- If there is a preponderance of loose, sagging, excess fat in the neck, Botox can only do so much. Surgical treatment is absolutely recommended in most cases.

- Face-lifts are designed to pick up, clean up, and crisp up the jawline and neck. A face-lift indicator is from the mouth down. Face-lifts work best with drooping jowls and loose skin under the chin.

Here's where I believe cosmetic surgery should be the last resort, if that:

- Drooping forehead. I don't believe in brow lifts. Nearly all of my patients who think they need a brow lift actually *don't* need one. For them, Botox does the trick. I've treated hundreds of patients who've had brow lifts, with a painful recuperation, only to see the drooping return within a year.

- Face-lifts to replace lost volume.

One of the biggest misconceptions about face-lifts is that they're all you need to look younger. People think they need to be stretched and tightened when in truth they need to be plumped. You don't want to pull too much because a rounded face in the bloom of youth is not pulled, it's full. So I always say the ideal is reestablishing youthful contours.

Face-lifts are also *not* intended to be a treatment for lines and wrinkles. They do absolutely nothing for overall fine wrinkling, uneven pigmentation, or a loss of radiance. They may soften a few of the naso-labial folds (lines between your nose and lips) or the marionette lines (from your lips down to your chin), but they aren't designed to eliminate them entirely. If your skin were pulled tightly enough to remove all of these lines, you would look quite bizarre. Furthermore, due to the initial post-operative swelling, the naso-labial folds might look much better, but once your face has settled and the swelling goes down, the lines will return—usually in about six months or so. Fillers and lasers are a much better choice for these kinds of lines and folds.

Now, if you start taking care of your skin at a younger age, and have regular visits to the dermatologist for fillers, you may not get to that point where surgery would be recommended at all. Given the number of faces I've seen and treated, I do think there are too many *repeat* face-lifts. Often, one is enough. The changes that do occur over time after the face-lift can often be treated nonsurgically. (Botox can work on muscles and fillers can fix some of the droopiness.) I can't tell you how many times I've seen patients literally transformed simply with a few needles. A skilled dermatologist can often effect more of a change than a face-lift could have done.

Bear this in mind as you research what procedures are available and might be recommended. That's where a regular regimen of maintenance is so important in the long run. You may be spared the risks involved with any surgical procedure, which is especially important for smokers and diabetics, who don't heal well. (Yet another reason to not eat sugar!) Or you may have specific types of sagging skin that will respond well to surgery. If that's the case, then I say go for it!

Fortunately, I have the kind of practice where most of my patients are more than content with the noninvasive procedures I can provide. From my experience, I think the trend is shifting away from surgery. It hurts. It has inherent risks. A certain recuperation time is mandatory. There can be complications and unforeseen side effects. And so many of my patients remark about the truly terrible work they've seen their friends or acquaintances endure—work that often can't be undone. That's enough to keep them adamant that surgery will only be a last resort for them.

If you are contemplating surgery, and if you are a good candidate for it, ask your dermatologist and trusted friends for referrals of competent surgeons board certified by the American Board of Plastic Surgery. You should see at least two or three different surgeons, ask all of them the same questions, and write down their recommendations. Weigh who says what. Look at their before and after photographs closely. Some surgeons are known for specific techniques or shaping; Doctor X might give all his patients the "same" nose, for example. Be sure to ascertain who is doing the procedure. Prominent surgeons with busy practices often do only some of the surgical work, then hand off the final stitching to their junior associates.

Most of all, you have to like the surgeon, like his staff, feel safe with his ideas and his aesthetic. Don't feel pressured. If you're not sure, don't do it. You can always reschedule. And if you go to see a cosmetic surgeon to discuss your drooping eyelids and he ends up telling you that you need six different procedures, including cheek and chin implants, I wouldn't hesitate to walk right out the door.

Remember, plastic surgery can do wonderful things with the right patient—and the right surgeon.

PART III

The 10 Minutes/ 10 Years Solution System

IN THIS PART, each chapter will describe different aging concerns and problems, and how to treat them, using the list of treatments introduced in the preceding chapter. (If a certain problem is not applicable to a specific category, it will not be listed.) I suggest you read through each section before deciding which products and/or treatments might suit you best. You won't need all of them. Discuss your needs with your dermatologist. Everyone has different skin-care needs.

Where applicable, there will be simple steps for a skin-care routine that can be done in 10 minutes or less. Don't forget: Anyone starting a specific skin-care regimen should see some results in a month. (After all, you can't undo a lifetime of skin abuse overnight.) But only by sticking to a new regimen religiously and as directed for *at least twelve weeks* will you begin to see *profound* results.

Treatments from Least to Most Intensive

Over-the-Counter (OTC) Skin-Care Products

Prescription Topicals

Mechanical Exfoliation

Intense Pulsed Light, GentleWaves LED, Photodynamic Therapy, Coblation, Thermage, and Titan

Injectible Fillers

Muscle Freezers

Chemical Peels

Lasers

5

Wrinkles

"CAN YOU BELIEVE IT? Just look at me! Look at these things on my face! They're *huge!*" Jodie exclaimed as soon as I walked into the examination room where she sat waiting, her cheeks flushed and her eyes full of tears.

From the near-hysteria in her voice, I fully expected to see a melanoma growing on Jodie's cheeks. Fortunately, there was no cancerous spot. There were hardly any spots at all. Jodie was in the bloom of health, her cheeks smooth and unlined.

"Look!" she said again, now pointing to her eyes. "Crow's-feet! Oh, God, I look just like my mother! You've just got to help me!"

Now, Jodie was overreacting just a bit. She had the barest hint of crow's-feet. And—she was only twenty-five. But for her, the appearance of a few tiny new lines was evidence enough that an appropriate skin-care regimen wasn't something she could ignore any longer.

Most of my patients aren't quite as upset or as obsessive as Jodie about their faces—and certainly not at twenty-five—but they're certainly not happy about wrinkles, either. Some of them who have marvelous skin and beautiful bone structure panic about lines that, frankly, only they can see in what they claim is certain light, or in their rearview mirrors when they're driving. Or small lines of expression that come with happy, animated faces. Part of this obsession stems from the social double standard women face: that it's okay for men to age normally, but women have to maintain that illusion of youth till their faces are practically frozen into wrinkle-free, super-stretched masks. It's disheartening, certainly, when beautiful, vital, normally aging women despair over their wrinkles and try everything they can to look like teenagers again.

It doesn't make them feel much better when I tell them that every woman, no matter how scrupulous she is about skin care and sun protection, starts to see very subtle changes by her late twenties or early thirties. By the time my patients come in, I often hear them lament, "All of a sudden, I woke up and saw wrinkles all over the place. Help!" I reassure them that no one ages overnight. The changes occur very subtly, over time—it's more like a creeping progression. The reason you notice is the lines become deep enough or the defect becomes severe enough to suddenly seem to "pop."

No other telltale sign of aging is as visible as fine lines and wrinkles. Despite the astonishing advances we've made in the last decade in terms of tackling and being able to erase and minimize these fine lines and wrinkles, there's still no magic potion that will keep them at bay forever.

Wrinkles are defined as ridges or creases on a surface—in this case, on the surface of the skin. They're triggered by an inflammatory response to some form of damage in the lower levels of the epidermis. When this damage is repeatedly repaired on a microscopic level, eventually it results in a visible line.

While some wrinkles are the result of repetitive muscle movement, such as frown lines and smile lines, the overwhelming majority of fine lines, wrinkles, and creases are due solely to photo-aging. Go out in the sun and start to count your wrinkles!

I always tell my patients that they can spend as much as they want to on expensive treatments over the years, but the easiest, cheapest, and least invasive way to prevent and minimize future wrinkles is to apply a broad-spectrum UVA/UVB–blocking sunscreen 365 days a year. Hundreds of patients come in and tell me about the $300 night repair creams they're using, but if they don't pair that with daily, repeated use of sunscreen, they might as well just tear up their money and throw it out the window. It does drive me a little crazy when the patients I see in my Miami office swear they use sunscreen religiously, even when their skin has been baked to a crispy, crunchy brown and is dotted with hyperpigmentation spots (which I'll discuss in chapter 6). These same patients plead for help, happily undergo multiple treatments, then go right back out in the sun and undo everything I've done!

Fredric Brandt, MD

So don't even think about serious treatment of wrinkles unless you're serious about staying out of the sun.

All wrinkles are not created equal. They're classified as shallow, fine, or superficial; or coarse, medium, or deep, which are more like furrows or creases. Superficial wrinkles should *not* be treated the same way as medium-depth or deep wrinkles and folds. They respond well to the least invasive treatments. But bear in mind that someone with superficial wrinkles may not have deep wrinkles, but I've yet to treat a patient with deep wrinkles who didn't also have superficial wrinkles.

This is an important concept, as the most common dermatological treatment for wrinkles is Botox, followed by injectible fillers. All fillers are not created equal, either. Your doctor should be suggesting a varied regimen to treat the various depths of wrinkles on your face. This is called tissue tailoring, and it's where the skill of your dermatologist is crucial. If he or she tells you that one filler fits all, then I suggest you say thank you and walk out the door!

1. FINE, OR SUPERFICIAL WRINKLES

Over-the-Counter (OTC) Skin-Care Products

Scan the shelves in the cosmetic aisles in your local department store and your head will start spinning. The care and treatment of wrinkles is cause, I believe, for the greatest amount of hype. While every woman needs a good moisturizer and a wrinkle treatment cream, you can be discriminating in your selection. No OTC cream can have the same profound effect as an injectible filler such as Restylane, or a muscle paralyzer, such as Botox or Reloxin. OTC wrinkle creams can soften and improve the appearance of fine lines and wrinkles, and provide the immediate benefit of hydrating the skin. OTC wrinkle creams *cannot* physically eliminate deeper lines. Only an injected substance can do that. Heavy problems need heavy hitters!

That doesn't mean, of course, that you shouldn't maintain your skin at home with daily use of wrinkle creams. Injectible fillers and OTC products are not mutually exclusive—they're complementary. No matter what you decide to do to treat deeper wrinkles, you'll still want to treat your skin to prevent preexisting wrinkles from getting worse and preventing as many new ones as possible from forming. In addition, you want to use your sunscreen to prevent any wrinkles from getting worse.

MOISTURIZERS

A moisturizer's function is to hydrate the skin. It is not designed to treat wrinkles. Don't believe any extravagant wrinkle-busting claims—because they aren't believable!

Use moisturizers in the morning and at night, as needed.

Moisturizers

Dr. Brandt Infinite Moisture

Dr. Brandt Poreless Moisture

Kinerase Cream

M.D. Forté Replenish Hydrating Cream

MD Skincare Hydra-Pure Intense Moisture Cream

ANTI-AGING/WRINKLE CREAMS: ALPHA HYDROXY ACIDS (AHA), ANTI-OXIDANTS, COLLAGEN PROMOTERS, AND PEPTIDES

Choose one or a combination of the following categories. While it's okay to layer different products with different functions, do not use more than four at a time (not counting cleanser and toner), as you can cause irritation and breakouts. See the sample treatment on page 124 for suggestions.

Remember that although these products feel like moisturizers, they are *treatment* creams. If you apply one in the morning, the correct application order is treatment cream, then moisturizer, then sunscreen. (Sunscreen is mandatory, as you will get burned and more wrinkled otherwise!) Let each layer be completely absorbed before adding another one.

Alpha-Hydroxy Acids/AHA Creams

Anakiri Transformation Eye and Neck Serum

Cellex-C Betaplex Smooth Skin Complex

Dr. Brandt V-Zone Neck Cream

M.D. Forté Facial Cream II or III

Z. Bigatti Re-storation Skin Treatment

Anti-Oxidants

Dr. Brandt C-Gel

Dr. Brandt Lineless Cream

Physician's Complex C-Plus Anti-Oxidant Serum

Prevage

SkinMedica Dermal Repair Cream

Topix Replenix Cream or Serum

Collagen Promoters

DDF Retinol Energizing Moisturizer

Dr. Brandt Contour Effect

SkinCeuticals Retinol 1.0

SkinMedica Retinol Complex

Peptide Creams

Dr. Brandt R3P Cream

Kinerase C6 Peptide Invasive Treatment

Physician's Complex Peptide Cream

122

10 MINUTES / 10 YEARS

WRINKLE RELAXERS AND TEXTURE IMPROVEMENT

Wrinkle Relaxers

Bliss Crease Police

Caudalie Lifting Serum

DERMAdoctor Immobile Lines Instant Topical Line Relaxer

Dr. Brandt Crease Release

Texture Improvement Creams

Cellex-C Betaplex Line Smoother

Dior Capture Serum

Dr. Brandt Liquid Skin

Juvena Rejuven Q10

Prescription Topicals

Tretinoin (the active ingredient in Renova and Retin-A) and tazarotene (the active ingredient in Avage and Tazorac) are the only skin-care ingredients FDA-approved for the treatment of fine wrinkles. Unless it causes severe irritation—and it shouldn't if used as prescribed, as there are many formulations; your dermatologist can try to find the one best suited to your skin's sensitivity level—a retinoid is a fantastic wrinkle treatment for everyone.

Always apply a retinoid *only* to dry skin, as it's far less irritating than when applied to damp or wet skin.

Retinoids substantially increase susceptibility to sunburn. For some of my patients, getting a terrible, peeling burn on their faces because they "forgot" to put on their sunscreen yet again is the only way to make them realize quite how badly they abuse their skin and how they need to protect it more than ever.

Mechanical Exfoliation

I recommend a series of microdermabrasion treatments for superficial wrinkles. It will definitely help. For best results, go once a month for four months, repeated every year, if needed.

Intense Pulsed Light, GentleWaves LED, Photodynamic Therapy, Coblation, Thermage, and Titan

Try either IPL, GentlesWaves LED, or Coblation for fine lines and wrinkles.

Injectible Fillers

Use *only* fillers designated for fine lines, as the others would be overkill. That means either CosmoDerm (collagen) or Restylane Fine Lines (hyaluronic acid).

Muscle Freezers

Botox or Reloxin can be used to treat fine lines, but only in the deftest hands.

Chemical Peels

Very superficial and superficial peels effectively treat superficial wrinkles. Try a series of four treatments—once every six weeks during the course of one year.

Lasers

Stick to the non-ablative lasers for superficial wrinkles—either CoolTouch, Smoothbeam, NLite, Gemini, or Fraxel.

10-Minute Regimen

My philosophy is to attack wrinkles with a two-tiered OTC approach: prevent and repair. First, you prevent them with a restructuring treatment cream, to help prevent the degradation of collagen. That's followed by the more immediate gratification of a wrinkle-relaxing cream, which temporarily repairs the wrinkle and also has a cumulative effect over time as it relaxes the musculature.

Before You Start

- Always cleanse before applying product. Use toner if you like, as well as an eye cream.

- Morning regimens must include use of a broad-spectrum sunscreen of your choice.

- For best results, always follow product instructions *exactly* as listed.

  For a woman with some sun damage, normal skin, and superficial wrinkles.

A.M.: Preventative

1. Cleanser, toner, eye cream.

2. Anti-aging serum: prevents and repairs glycation, gives anti-oxidant boost, protects against free-radical damage.

3. Sunscreen.

P.M.: Repair

1. Cleanser, toner, eye cream.

2. Peptide cream: to stimulate collagen production and promote cellular renewal while replenishing moisture. Apply every other night for the first two weeks in order to avoid dry, flaky skin; then every night thereafter.

3. Moisturizing treatment: to hydrate skin.

Special Treatments

Home Microdermabrasion: Polishes complexion while improving overall texture of skin. Gently massage on damp skin for two minutes; rinse. Use twice a week, leaving three to four days between treatments.

Home Peel: tightens pores, improves firmness, and brightens skin. Follow instructions in kits. Use every ten days. Never use on the same day as home microdermabrasion.

2. MEDIUM-DEPTH WRINKLES

The treatment of medium wrinkles necessitates slightly more invasive procedures.

Over-the-Counter (OTC) Skin-Care Products

Prescription Topicals

Mechanical Exfoliation

Follow the same regimen as for superficial wrinkles, as skin still needs to be hydrated, repaired, and protected. Bear in mind that OTC products, retinoids, and microdermabrasion will have less of an effect on medium wrinkles and should not be expected to perform as well as fillers can.

Injectible Fillers

Fillers are ideal for medium wrinkles. They will give you visible results and replace lost volume. The best fillers for the mid-dermis are ArteFill, CosmoPlast, Restylane, Hylaform and Hylaform Plus, Juvéderm, Perlane, Sculptra, and fat transfer, often done in some combination. I often use Restylane with an overlay of CosmoDerm to complete the correction.

Muscle Freezers

Botox and Reloxin will definitely soften medium-depth wrinkles.

Chemical Peels

For medium wrinkles, a medium peel is the best. It can be done with TCA, Jessner's solution, or a combination of Jessner's solution and glycolic acid. Discuss your options with your dermatologist.

Lasers

Most people should still stick to non-ablative lasers: CoolTouch, Smoothbeam, NLite, or Gemini. Fraxel will also work. For a proliferation of fine wrinkles on crepey skin, you may want to consider the Erbium:YAG laser.

10-Minute Regimen

For a woman with sun damage, loss of resiliency, normal skin, and medium wrinkles.

A.M.: Preventative

1. Cleanser, toner, eye cream.

2. Wrinkle relaxer: relaxes stress and tension on muscles, diminishing appearance of fine lines and wrinkles.

3. Anti-aging serum: prevents and repairs glycation, gives anti-oxidant boost, protects against free-radical damage.

4. Skin tightener: tightens and firms skin.

5. Sunscreen.

P.M.: Repair

1. Cleanser, toner, eye cream.

2. Anti-aging cream: to stimulate collagen production and promote cellular renewal while replenishing moisture. Apply every other night for the first two weeks to avoid dry, flaky skin; then every night thereafter.

3. Moisturizing treatment: to hydrate skin.

Special Treatments

Home Microdermabrasion: polishes complexion while improving overall texture of skin. Gently massage on damp skin for two minutes; rinse. Use twice a week, leaving three to four days between treatments.

Home Peel: Tightens pores, improves firmness, and brightens skin. Follow instructions in kits. Use every ten days. Never use on the same day as home microdermabrasion.

3. DEEP WRINKLES

Deep wrinkles need deep intervention. While topical creams can have a softening effect, more serious intervention is usually required. As with superficial and medium wrinkles, deep wrinkles are caused by photo-aging and mechanical repetitive use over the years—who wants to stop smiling?—but also are due to lost volume in the face. As such, they're more like folds and creases than lines, and will respond only to volume replacement in the form of fillers, or serious peels and lasers that target the deepest layers of skin. In other words, what will work best is to not only fill the wrinkle, but to add volume to the face to lift the wrinkle as well.

Over-the-Counter (OTC) Skin-Care Products

Prescription Topicals

Follow the guidelines for superficial wrinkles, but don't expect them to disappear, as it's physiologically impossible.

Mechanical Exfoliation

Microdermabrasion will not alter deep wrinkles and folds. You may want to consider dermabrasion, but *only* if your dermatologist has years of experience and you're prepared for the pain and recuperation period.

Injectible Fillers

Fillers are a must for deep wrinkles. The best fillers for the deeper dermis are ArteFill, CosmoPlast, Restylane, Hylaform and Hylaform Plus, Juvéderm, Sculptra, and fat transfer, often done in some combination.

Muscle Freezers

Botox or Reloxin should be used in conjunction with fillers.

Chemical Peels

A deep chemical peel will have a visible effect on deep wrinkles, but it is a painful process with a lengthy recuperation period.

Lasers

A CO_2 laser will also have a remarkable effect on deep wrinkles, but it too is a painful process with a lengthy recuperation period.

10-Minute Regimen

For a woman with sun damage, dry skin, loss of resiliency, and deep wrinkles.

A.M.: Preventative

1. Cleanser, toner, eye cream.

2. Wrinkle relaxer: relaxes stress and tension on muscles, diminishing appearance of fine lines and wrinkles.

3. Anti-aging collagen promoter: stimulates collagen; hydrates for plumper-looking skin.

4. Sunscreen.

P.M.: Repair

1. Cleanser, toner, eye cream.

2. Anti-aging cream: to stimulate collagen production and promote cellular renewal while replenishing moisture (if you're using AHAs or retinols). Apply every other night for the first two weeks to avoid dry, flaky skin; then every night thereafter.

3. Moisturizing treatment: to hydrate skin.

Special Treatments

Home Microdermabrasion: polishes complexion while improving overall texture of skin. Gently massage on damp skin for two minutes; rinse. Use twice a week, leaving three to four days between treatments.

Home Peel: tightens pores, improves firmness, and brightens skin. Follow instructions in kits. Use every ten days. Never use on the same day as home microdermabrasion.

10-Minute Tips

- Between steps in your skin-care regimen: choose your outfit, make some coffee, feed the cat—you'll see that each step goes by in a flash. Every regimen listed should take under 10 minutes to apply.

- Sun damage causes wrinkles. Protect yourself every day!

- Always apply gels or serums before lotions or creams.

- If you're in a rush, use your hair dryer on "cold" to dry skin-care products more quickly, so you can go on to the next step!

- To avoid irritation, don't get too close to your lashes when applying eye creams.

- Keep your fingers away from your face during the day.

- Take care not to make too many overly animated facial expressions.

- While it's next to impossible to not move around while sleeping, try to fall asleep on your back, to avoid crushing your face into the pillow.

- Stay away from secondhand smoke.

- See the tips in chapters 1 and 2 for more suggestions.

Before

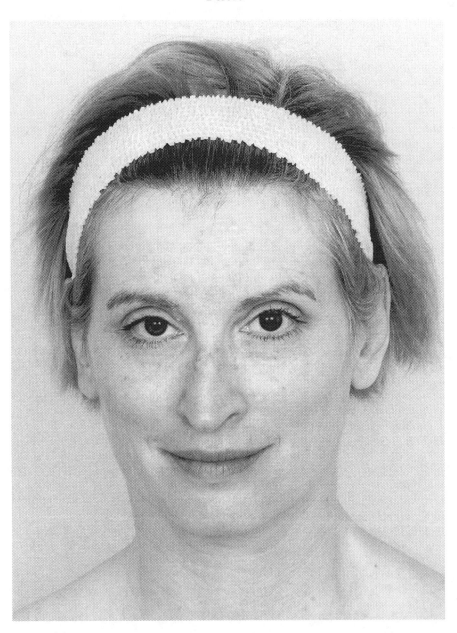

Fredric Brandt, MD

After

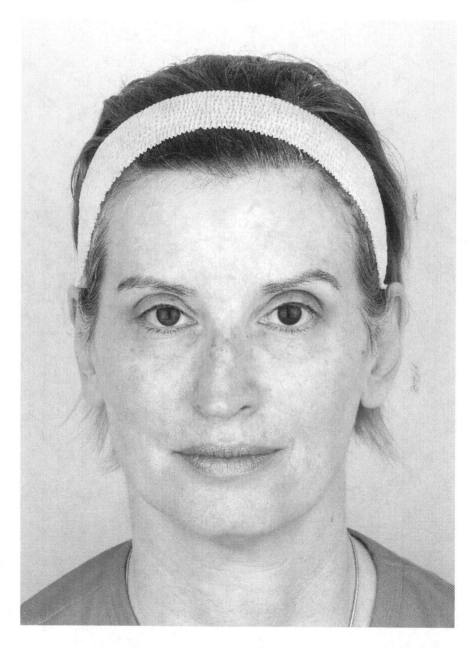

Botox in the furrows (between the brows), crow's-feet, and neck.
Restylane in the cheeks, lips, and jawline, and under the eyes. Collagen around the lips.

Before

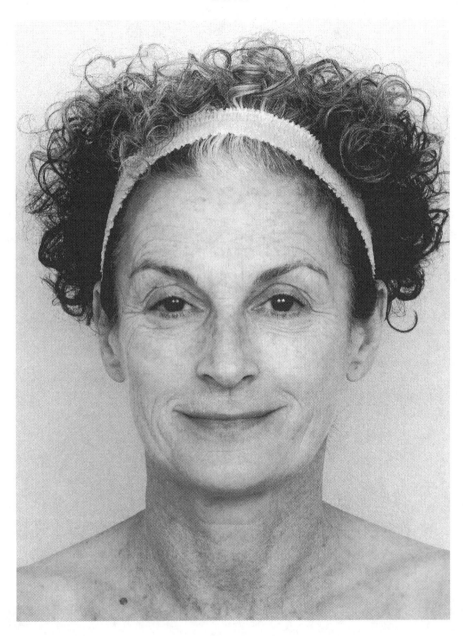

Fredric Brandt, MD

After

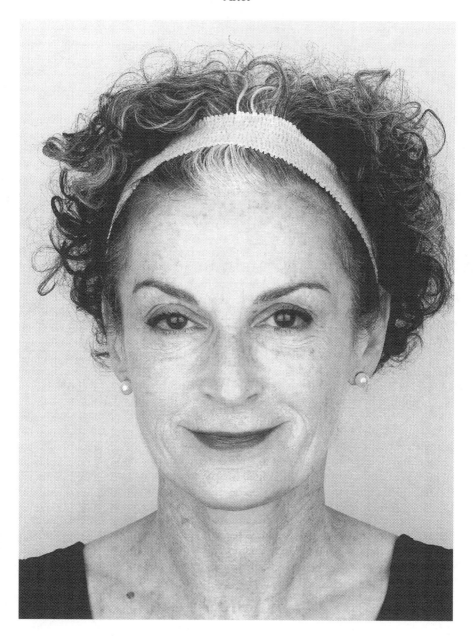

Botox in the furrows (between the brows), crow's-feet, and neck.
Restylane in the cheeks, lips, and jawline, and under the eyes. Collagen around the lips.

6

Hyperpigmentation and Hypopigmentation

HYPERPIGMENTATION, OR *DYSCHROMIA*, is a general term for an increased, abnormal production of the pigment called melanin that creates spots or blotchiness and uneven skin tone. When the melanin-producing cells called melanocytes are damaged, they increase in size. This phenomenon is triggered by several factors: sun exposure, response to inflammation as with acne, or a hormonal factor.

When skin is exposed to the sun, the resulting spots are usually red or brown—they're freckles (solar lentigos), or age or liver spots. (They have nothing to do with your liver, except to resemble it in color!) Frankly, they shouldn't be called age spots—they should be called sun spots, because too much solar radiation is directly responsible for creating them.

Hyperpigmentation that's a result of inflammation, as with healing acne pimples or pustules, is called post-inflammatory hyperpigmentation. Those with fair skin might start out seeing red or purplish-red spots that gradually turn brown before fading. People of color might see the spots turn dark brown or blackish before fading—a process that can often take many long months.

Hormonal changes in women can also cause hyperpigmentation. When that happens, triggered by pregnancy, birth control pills, perimenopause, or menopause, it's called *melasma*. I'll discuss melasma in more detail on page 144.

Rarely, certain types of solar lentigos can become *lentigo maligna melanoma*, a form of skin cancer. Of course, you know by now that you should have a full-body check for spots and skin cancer every year, but if you notice a sudden proliferation of any type of spots, see a dermatologist to rule out any medical conditions.

Hyperpigmentation is incredibly common. Luckily, hyperpigmentation responds well to treatment—if and *only* if you commit to using sunscreen every day. Thinking you're protected simply by putting sunscreen with a high SPF on once in the morning is *not* enough to tackle this problem. You really need to think about altering your sun lifestyle. That means wearing hats, reapplying sunscreen every two hours, and becoming aware of how much casual sun exposure you get when you go outside, whether simply to run errands or to sit at a table outside for lunch.

Because most people are not aware of how often they must reapply sunscreen—or stay out of the sun altogether in order to treat pigmentation problems—they don't see results. They use repair creams or bleaching/lightening creams to fade sun damage, but undermine their efforts when they fail to protect their skin every day with a good broad-spectrum sunscreen. Instead of improving, they keep going in a vicious circle and wasting their time and money. They'll never get rid of spots because they aren't tackling the reason the spots are appearing in the first place! It takes less time for the sun to cause pigmentation problems than it does to create a tan.

Remember, you get sun damage through car windows, through glass, with indoor halogen lighting, and just by spending a few minutes outside every day. Lots of my patients who spend hours driving often have far more freckles and spots on their left side. Wonder why?

If you don't use sunscreen, you can undergo all the treatments for hyperpigmentation that you want, but the spots will quickly return with a vengeance.

As photo-aging destroys melanocytes over time, reverse freckles, or white spots, can also appear on the skin. This is called hypopigmentation, or *melanosis*. As no pigment is left in that area, the damage is irreversible.

Sometimes, hypopigmentation spots can develop growths called *stucco keratosis*. These need dermatologist treatment and removal, usually by freezing with liquid nitrogen. As these usually appear on the arms and legs, they're harder to treat than spots on the face. Skin on the face is the easiest to treat since it regenerates more quickly, thanks to its regular cell turnover as well as the preponderance of oil-producing sebaceous glands. The lower you go on the body, the harder skin problems are to treat and the longer they take to heal.

1. NON-HORMONAL HYPERPIGMENTATION

Over-the-Counter (OTC) Skin-Care Products

Hyperpigmentation is one of the few skin conditions that responds extremely well to simple OTC treatment. Most of the products available are called skin whiteners, lighteners, or bleachers. Using one of these products will *not* make your skin white or turn you into Michael Jackson. All they can do is gently retard or block the production of melanin you already have from coming to the surface of the skin, preventing spots from forming. As such, they're safe to use, no matter what your skin tone.

The most commonly used ingredient in American whiteners and bleachers is hydroquinone, sold OTC in up to a 2 percent concentration. Other approved ingredients include arbutin, kojic acid, and licorice extract.

Although hydroquinone has been tested and used for decades in America, it is not approved for use in many other countries in the world. In August 2006, the FDA proposed a ban on OTC use of hydroquinone, claming it is a possible carcinogen, so it remains to be seen if the ban will be upheld.

Hydroquinone blocks your melanin, and ingredients such as albatin, which blocks the activity of the enzyme tyrosinase, responsible for triggering melanin synthesis, work instead by preventing melanin's formation in the first place. Cleanser, toner, day lotion, night cream, and serum are available without hydroquinone in Asia, where women tend to stay out of the sun and take the concept of skin lightening seriously. There are now similar lines of products available in America.

Ideally, you should begin seeing visible results in days from any bleaching/lightening product. Bear in mind that "visible" doesn't mean a dramatic shift from black to white or from brown to white. Instead, you should see a general improvement to your overall skin tone as well as a gradual fading of freckles and spots.

Which brings me to a crucial point: From the research we've done, far too many consumers do not understand what exactly a bleaching/lightening product can do. They think it will bleach out spots on skin the way chlorine bleach rids clothing of spots and stains. OTC brighteners/lighteners are not spot treatments. They must be used over the entire face. And if the hyperpigmentation spots are very dark, they may not respond to any OTC treatments at all. (See the section on lasers on page 142.) And, of course, *no* brightening will happen unless you use your sunscreen.

Remember that these lightening products are meant to be integrated into your daily regimen; they aren't replacements for other treatment creams. Use a lightener, then a treatment cream, then a moisturizer, and sunscreen comes last. Allow each layer to be completely absorbed before adding another one. Never use more than four products (excluding cleanser and toner) at a time.

You can also try using OTC creams that contain vitamin A, vitamin A, and/or soy, as these all have a mild spot-lightening effect.

You can also speed the lightening process along by using home peels and home microdermabrasion, or a complete lightening regimen. Their exfoliating properties will allow the active ingredients in the lighteners to penetrate more effectively.

Lighteners/Brighteners

B. Kamins Skin Lightening Treatment

Cellex-C Fade Away Gel

Clarins Bright Plus Total Brightening Serum

Dr. Brandt Laser Lightning Serum

Dr. Brandt Laser Lightning System

Home Microdermabrasion

B. Kamins Microdermabrasion Kit

Dr. Brandt Microdermabrasion

Neutrogena Advanced Solutions At Home MicroDermabrasion System

Olay Regenerist Microdermabrasion and Peel System

Home Peels

Dr. Brandt Laser A-Peel

Lancôme Resurface Peel

MD Skincare Alpha Beta Daily Face Peel

Prescription Topicals

Hydroquinone is available in a stronger concentration, 4 percent, by prescription. It's also often combined in prescription with either one of the retinoids or with glycolic acid. In addition, a strong concentration of glycolic acid will also fade hyperpigmentation spots.

Mechanical Exfoliation

Microdermabrasion will help fade spots. At least one course over several months, if not more, will be needed.

Intense Pulsed Light, GentleWaves LED, Photodynamic Therapy, Coblation, Thermage, and Titan

Try either IPL, GentleWaves, Photodynamic Therapy, or Titan. A series may have to be repeated.

Coblation and Thermage are not intended to treat hyperpigmentation.

Chemical Peels

A dermatologist can do either a light peel with salicylic acid, glycolic acid, TCA, or Jessner's peels, or a medium TCA or glycolic acid combination peel. A series may be needed. A deep peel is not recommended.

Lasers

Lasers can work wonders on hyperpigmentation, as the pigment lasers are specifically designed to target brown spots. Best for those are the Q-switched ruby, the Q-switched alexandrite, the Q-switched Nd:YAG, and the Aura lasers. You can also use the Gemini laser in the 532 mode, as well as Fraxel. For serious cases, you might want to consider the Erbium:YAG or the CO_2 laser.

10-Minute Regimen

For a woman with hyperpigmentation. It's essential to follow this regimen consistently, twice a day, every day. Never leave home without sunscreen on!

A.M.: Preventative

1. Cleanser, toner, eye cream.

2. Skin lightener/brightener: evens out skin tone and brightens dull skin. Use a serum or lotion.

3. Anti-oxidant cream: anti-oxidant boost, protects against free-radical damage.

4. Sunscreen.

P.M.: Repair

1. Cleanser, toner, eye cream.

2. Skin lightener/brightener: evens out skin tone and brightens dull skin. Use a serum or lotion.

3. Anti-aging cream: protects and prevents depletion of collagen while preserving moisture and elasticity of the skin.

4. Moisturizing treatment: to hydrate skin.

Special Treatments

Home Microdermabrasion: polishes complexion while improving overall texture of skin. Gently massage on damp skin for two minutes; rinse. Use twice a week, leaving three to four days between treatments.

Home Peel: tightens pores, improves firmness, and brightens skin. Follow instructions in kits. Use every ten days. Never use on the same day as home microdermabrasion.

TREATMENT FOR PRECANCEROUS SPOTS

If your dermatologist determines that you have precancerous spots, you'll need treatment with prescription creams more potent than anything available OTC. Commonly prescribed is Solaraze, an aspirin-derivative cream applied twice a day for about three to six months. It gradually removes some precancerous spots without much downtime, but it's not quite as effective as some of the more aggressive treatments. For stubborn cases, you can try Carac or Aldara, which are topical immune response modifiers. You'll need to use them for several weeks. During that time, the spots will peel and look pretty bad, and then eventually slough off altogether.

Photodynamic Light Therapy can also be effective, as well as a CO_2 laser.

2. HORMONAL HYPERPIGMENTATION: MELASMA

I've seen many pregnant patients over the years. Most are beaming with happiness and that certain pregnancy glow. But others are not quite as glowing, as they've developed brown spots and irregularly shaped blotches on their faces, often called the "Pregnancy Mask," that can cause acute embarrassment and shame. This is the legacy of melasma.

Melasma can look the same as sun-induced hyperpigmentation, but because it's hormonal in nature, it's much tougher to treat. It usually doesn't respond as well to OTC lighteners as non-hormonal hyperpigmentation does. For some unknown reason, melasma is like a bad memory—one that keeps coming back to haunt you. Sometimes it fades on its own after pregnancy, but sometimes it doesn't. It can be very stressful for older women whose perimenopausal symptoms affect the quality of their lives.

Melasma will never improve unless you take great pains to always shield your skin from the sun. Don't just use sunscreen, but get used to hats and complete sun avoidance during the peak exposure hours of 10 a.m. to 4 p.m. I always tell my patients that they alone are responsible for making a choice: If they want to be tan, they will never get rid of their melasma, and it's not worth prescribing treatments or procedures if they aren't willing to do their part.

Sometimes confused with melasma is *Favre-Racouchot syndrome*, triggered by years of sun damage and smoking that leads to the formation of large comedones (blackheads) around the eyes and upper cheeks. A dermatologist will treat them with topical retinoids and/or surgical extraction.

Over-the Counter (OTC) Skin-Care Products

Follow the suggestions for non-hormonal hyperpigmentation. If you use home peels, use them once a week.

Prescription Topicals

The 4 percent concentration of hydroquinone (often in the non-micronized form, such as EpiQuin) is usually combined with a retinoid, such as Retin-A, as well as a cortisone cream such as Tri-Luma. It can also be combined with a glycolic acid like Lustra-Ultra, or with a retinoid like Lustra-AF. Discuss your options with your dermatologist.

Many of these drugs cannot be used if you are pregnant or breast-feeding. Always talk to your obstetrician about any prescription medication prior to taking it.

Mechanical Exfoliation

Intense Pulsed Light, GentleWaves LED, Photodynamic Therapy, Coblation, Thermage, and Titan

Follow the recommendations for non-hormonal hyperpigmentation.

Chemical Peels

Chemical peels for melasma are controversial. A series of light peels that might work well on non-hormonal hyperpigmentation might *not* work for melasma. In addition, there are different skin types, as classified on the Fitzpatrick list (see page 22 in chapter 2). Those who are Type I and Type II, with very fair skin, respond best to peels for melasma. But for Type III through Type VI skin types, the likelihood is high that they may become red and inflamed, leading ironically to the development of non-hormonal post-inflammatory hyperpigmentation! For them, any intensive procedure may trigger more pigmentation changes.

If you do have melasma and you do not have fair skin, you need to have a

146146

146 # 146

146# 146

146

146146

146

146## 146

146

146# 146

146

146

146

146

146

146

146

146

Fredric Brandt, MD

- Peels or microdermabrasion take off the barrier layer of dead skin cells, making you more susceptible to burns. Never go out in the sun after any of these procedures without sunscreen.

- Retinols and retinoids also increase sun sensitivity. There's no point in taking the time and trouble to treat your skin for hyperpigmentation if you aren't willing to take the 10 minutes to adequately protect your skin from the sun at all times.

7

Loss of Radiance and Dull, Dry, Blotchy Skin

"MY SKIN JUST LOOKS SO — I don't know, what's the word? — *blah,*" said Tracy, a new patient of thirty-eight, told me. "It's dull and blotchy, and it makes me look a lot older than I really am. You can tell me what to do, right?"

Tracy needed to get her glow back. As we get older, the skin-cell turnover gradually starts to slow, resulting in more dead skin cells of the stratum corneum accumulating on the surface. Skin loses its radiance and translucency. Too much sun exposure and, especially, smoking those cigarettes will also give skin a sallow, dull tone. The key to waking up blah skin is to clean out the pores, increase skin-cell turnover, regenerate collagen, and brighten and polish the skin's surface when you exfoliate, exfoliate, exfoliate. You also need to make sure your skin is properly hydrated, because skin that is plumped up with moisture automatically looks a lot better. (An easy adjunct is to humidify your home. Even if you live in the tropics, air-conditioning sucks moisture out of the air, leaving your home as dry as a desert.)

As with hyperpigmentation, dealing with a loss of radiance can easily be treated with OTC products. In fact, products designed to treat this—with "radiance" and "luminosity" on the label—are proliferating, which means that cosmetics companies have recognized that consumers are looking for help. The heart of all "de-blah" regimens is home microdermabrasion and peeling. Alternate home microdermabrasion with home peels, and be sure to combine them with a treatment cream that speeds up cell turnover rate.

If your skin is blotchy, try the hyperpigmentation regimen on page 142 in chapter 6, or see the sections on redness in chapter 20.

Over-the-Counter (OTC) Skin-Care Products

Moisturizers

Dr. Brandt Infinite Moisture

Dr. Brandt Poreless Moisture

Kinerase Cream

M.D. Forté Replenish Hydrating Cream

MD Skincare Hydra-Pure Intense Moisture Cream

Anti-Aging Creams

Dr. Brandt Contour Effect Cream

Dr. Brandt Lineless Cream

Dr. Brandt R3P Cream

Kinerase C6 Peptide Invasive Treatment

SkinMedica Dermal Repair Cream

Home Microdermabrasion

If your skin is not sensitive and not too dry, or especially if you have oily skin, you can use a microdermabrasion cream up to twice a week. Those with normal or slightly dry skin can try once a week. If you're sensitive, stick to once every two weeks.

B. Kamins Microdermabrasion Kit

Dr. Brandt Microdermabrasion

Neutrogena Advanced Solutions At Home MicroDermabrasion System

Olay Regenerist Microdermabrasion and Peel System

Home Peels

As I said above, I believe that an ideal way to return radiance to the skin is to combine home peeling (chemical exfoliators) with home microdermabrasion (mechanical exfoliators). The active ingredients that tighten pores, improve overall firmness, and bring back the glow are glycolic and lactic acid. Start off peeling no more than once a week. Never do a peel on the same day as microdermabrasion. This can cause serious irritation.

Dr. Brandt Laser A-Peel

Lancôme Resurface Peel

Prescription Topicals

You can use any of the prescription retinoids.

Mechanical Exfoliation

Microdermabrasion is a definite yes, once every four weeks.

Intense Pulsed Light, GentleWaves LED, Photodynamic Therapy, Coblation, Thermage, and Titan

IPL or Photodynamic Therapy will wake up the skin. In addition, we have patients reporting that after a few treatments with the Titan, their complexions are improving. Even though the Titan is intended for tissue tightening, the intense infrared light and the resulting collagen stimulation might play a role in brightening the skin.

Chemical Peels

A series of four to six superficial TCA (trichloroacetic acid) peels will help exfoliate.

Lasers

Peeling lasers like the Erbium:YAG or the CO_2 will completely resurface blah skin, but with serious side effects. You might want to try Fraxel first.

10-Minute Regimen

For a woman with a loss of radiance and dull, blotchy skin.

This is the regimen I gave to Tracy. She started seeing results within two weeks and was very pleased with her progress as she continued to maintain this regimen.

A.M.: Preventative

1. Cleanser, toner, eye cream.

2. Lightening and brightening serum: to even out skin tone.

3. Anti-oxidant cream: anti-oxidant boost, protects against free-radical damage.

4. Sunscreen.

P.M.: Repair

1. Cleanser, toner, eye cream.

2. Lightening and brightening serum: to even out skin tone.

3. Anti-aging cream: to stimulate collagen production and promote cellular renewal while replenishing moisture (if you're using AHAs or retinols). Apply every other night for the first two weeks in order to avoid dry, flaky skin; then every night thereafter.

4. Moisturizing treatment: to hydrate skin.

Special Treatments

Home Microdermabrasion: polishes complexion while improving overall texture of skin. Gently massage on damp skin for two minutes; rinse. Use twice a week, leaving three to four days between treatments.

Home Peel: tightens pores, improves firmness, and brightens skin. Follow instructions in kits. Use every ten days. Never use on the same day as home microdermabrasion.

ABOUT DRY SKIN

Dryness is often misdiagnosed. There is truly dry skin or somewhat dry skin where you see dryness all over the face, which is usually due to loss of moisture content in the skin with age or with too much sun exposure (or both). This kind of dryness will respond to moisturizers. See the list on page 120 in chapter 5 for a comprehensive list of good moisturizers.

Often, however, patients will come in and say, "Oh, Dr. Brandt, my skin is so oily and I'm breaking out, but I'm dry at the same time. How can that be?" Or they'll say, "My skin is so sensitive. No matter what I put on it, it gets dry." Neither of these cases are really dryness—they're *inflammation*, properly called *seborrheic dermatitis*.

I can't tell you how important this distinction is. An overwhelming majority of my patients don't understand how common seborrheic dermatitis is. And unless that inflammation is treated, dryness (or other skin conditions, like acne) will not improve and may worsen. It is absolutely imperative that you not self-diagnose dryness. Let your dermatologist examine your skin and figure out the cause of your dryness so it can be appropriately treated.

Seborrheic dermatitis is caused when the oil (sebaceous) glands produce too much sebum, the natural oil you need to keep skin hydrated, which leads to the growth of the pityrosporum yeast that causes scaling, itching, dry patches, and flakes especially around the nose, eyebrows, the chin area, and the cheeks. On the scalp, it's often mistaken for dandruff. It may or may not go hand in hand with acne, which adds insult to injury for those who are already suffering from breakouts. Moisturizers alone are not a solution for seborrheic dermatitis.

The key to treating seborrheic dermatitis is reducing the irritation. I suggest trying OTC anti-redness or anti-inflammatory creams or lotions, as well as prescription creams such as Elidel, Protopic, or the new one called Atopiclair, a non-steroidal anti-inflammatory. It's best to stay away from the fluorinated prescription hydrocortisones, as these steroid creams can have side effects like thinning of the skin and broken blood vessels. If you are going to use a mild steroid cream on the face, make sure it's just a 0.5 percent to 1.0 percent hydrocortisone.

If you think you have truly sensitive skin, see chapter 20.

10-Minute Tips

- Loss of radiance responds very quickly to OTC treatment. Exfoliation takes only a minute or two. Make it a regular part of your skin-care regimen—and stick to it.

- Alternating between microdermabrasion and peels works well.

- Don't mistake dryness for irritation! Double-check with a dermatologist to be sure.

- Avoid extremes in climate—inside and out.

- Keep your skin and body hydrated. Decrease caffeine and alcohol consumption; drink lots of water; humidify your office and home.

- Be sure to stick to a hyperpigmentation regimen if you're using one.

8

Enlarged Pores

ONE OF THE COMPLAINTS I hear most often from my patients as they age is about the size of their pores. Sometimes, they tell me, it seems as though the pores are growing exponentially as they sleep! They can appear quite unsightly and trigger some very panicked reactions. But don't worry. Enlarged pores are common and respond well to OTC treatment.

Many people think that enlarged pores are a problem that comes with teenage acne and oily skin. That's true, of course, but as we age, our pores grow larger, too. With age, natural enlargement of the underlying oil (sebaceous) glands occurs, along with diminishment of collagen; consequently the ducts compress, allowing the oil glands to rise to the surface of the skin.

Enlarged pores often accompany the skin condition called *rosacea*. If you think you have rosacea, with its telltale trademark flush/blush response, please refer to chapter 20.

If you have enlarged pores, it's imperative to clean them out with the right cleanser and couple that with the use of the right treatment cream, preferably with salicylic acid, an anti-inflammatory ingredient that doesn't strip moisture from the skin while it cleans and clarifies. Don't forget that you can custom-tailor your cleansing routine—if you're up for it, as I realize that this is not exactly the most realistic suggestion! If you only have enlarged pores in the T-zone around the nose, cheeks, and forehead, try using a pore-specific cleanser there and use your regular cleanser on the rest of your face.

And stop scrubbing! Scrubbing won't minimize pores. It'll just make your skin dry, red, and irritated.

Over-the-Counter (OTC) Skin-Care Products

There are OTC products available that tackle enlarged pores. One of the advantages of using pore treatment creams and gels is that they are usually mattifying (oil-reducing) products. They'll cut down on oil production for those with oily skin, but work equally well to treat enlarged pores in those with dry skin, as they won't cause excessive dryness. And you can also layer them with other moisturizers or treatment creams that you regularly use for other skin concerns.

Many women with oily and/or combination skin are afraid to use any kind of moisturizer, fearful that they might clog their pores and intensify their tendency toward shininess. Don't starve your skin of hydration, though. Even if you have large pores and/or oily or combination skin, you still need to use a lightweight moisturizer. Look for a non-comedogenic, lightweight pore treatment containing salicylic acid, as well as tea tree oil to calm inflammation. (A side benefit is an anti-acne effect.) These products are ideal to use in the summer for all skin types, as some sunscreen can heat up the skin and cause more oil production.

If you use one of these products, you should begin to see some results right away. Pores will continue to be minimized the longer you use them.

A note about concealers: There are many concealers on the market that claim to minimize pores, but all they do is conceal (and sometimes magnify them into craters). They aren't treatments for enlarged pores and they don't do anything to reduce oil production. Try a pore-treatment gel or a skin smoother; their texture will help smooth the skin so that makeup will not sink down and make pores appear larger.

Pore Treatments

Clinique Pore Minimizer Instant Perfection

DERMAdoctor Picture Porefect Pore Minimizing Solution

Dr. Brandt Pore Effect Cream

Dr. Brandt Poreless Gel

Dr. Brandt Poreless Purifying Mask

Dr. Brandt Pores No More

Anti-Aging Creams

Retinols help increase the cell turnover rate, so the dead skin cells don't fall into the pores and clog them up.

Collagen Promoters/Retinols

Dr. Brandt "C"-Gel

SkinCeuticals Retinol 1.0

SkinMedica Retinol Complex

Texture Improvement Gels and Creams

Cellex-C Betaplex Line Smoother

Dior Capture Serum

Dr. Brandt Poreless Gel

Dr. Brandt Pores No More

Juvena Rejuven Q10

Home Microdermabrasion

This is a must to keep pores unclogged. Do it at least once or twice a week.

B. Kamins Microdermabrasion Kit

Dr. Brandt Microdermabrasion

Neutrogena Advanced Solutions At Home MicroDermabrasion System

Olay Regenerist Microdermabrasion and Peel Kit

Home Peels

Combine home peeling (chemical exfoliators) with home microdermabrasion (mechanical exfoliators). Start off peeling no more than once a week. Never do a peel on the same day as microdermabrasion to avoid serious irritation.

Dr. Brandt Laser A-Peel

Lancôme Resurface Peel

Prescription Topicals

A retinoid will help keep the pores unclogged so they look cleaner and smaller.

Mechanical Exfoliation

A course of microdermabrasion will also keep pores cleaned out.

Chemical Peels

Superficial chemical peels are best used to clean out debris in pores and help refine their appearance.

Lasers

Certain non-ablative lasers that heat deep into the skin will work wonders on enlarged pores. Especially the Smoothbeam and the Gemini, with the 10–64 component, where you're actually affecting the oil glands themselves and stimulating collagen production. This should definitely reduce the size of your pores.

10-Minute Regimen

For a woman with oily/combination skin and enlarged pores.

A.M.: Preventative

1. Cleanser, toner, eye cream. (Use a cleaner/toner to control excess oil while unclogging pores.)

2. Clarifying gel: to clean and refine pores, reduce oil production.

3. Pore treatment: mattifies shine and cleans and conceals pores; be sure to select one that treats the pores, not fills them in. (If your skin is oily, stick to pore-treatment gels. Those with combination skin will be better able to tolerate a cream.)

4. Sunscreen.

P.M.: Repair

1. Cleanser, toner, eye cream.

2. Clarifying gel: to clean and refine pores, reduce oil production. (If your skin is oily, use a lightweight moisturizer. Those with combination skin can try a slightly more substantial moisturizer.)

3. Pore treatment cream: clarifying, hydrating treatment that absorbs oil, unclogs pores, and calms redness.

Special Treatments

Home Microdermabrasion: polishes complexion while improving overall texture of skin. Gently massage on damp skin for two minutes; rinse. Use twice a week, leaving three to four days between treatments.

Home Peel: tightens pores, improves firmness, and brightens skin. Follow instructions in kits. Use every ten days. Never use on the same day as home microdermabrasion.

10-Minute Tips

- Do not scrub! Use a gentle cleanser.

- Stick to the regimen. Pores will be minimized with consistent use. These regimens should take you less than 10 minutes.

- Look for products with flaxseed to decrease the size of the sebaceous glands by reducing sebum production.

- Keep your collagen stimulated with OTC products such as retinols.

- Alternate between microdermabrasion and home peels for the best effect.

- Use sheer makeup that doesn't look cakey on your skin.

- If you think your hormones are out of whack and increasing oil production, see your gynecologist.

- During times of heightened stress, bodies produce more cortisol, which increases oil production. Dealing with stress should help your skin.

9

From the Eyebrows Up

LET'S TALK FOREHEADS. They can droop so dramatically that eyebrows descend over the eyes, giving people an unnaturally fierce expression. Your deadbeat boss who drives you to scowls or your innate tendency to frown when stressed or wrinkle your brow when laughing can cause lines, creases, and furrows. Over time, the lines become embedded into the skin once elasticity and resilience are lost. Skin that would have once snapped back loses its snap.

Most of which can be fixed by the wonder that is the botulinum toxin!

Botox and Reloxin have transformed the treatment of whatever's been etched into the skin of the forehead. They have a near-magical effect on mechanical lines and wrinkles caused by use of the underlying muscles. They can actually raise a drooping forehead. They can align uneven eyebrows.

In the right hands, of course. I'm pretty horrified by Botox's and Reloxin's continued misuse by those who inject it with the touch of a jackhammer. I see frozen foreheads devoid of any lines of expression when the rest of the face is aging slowly and gracefully. I've seen performers trying to emote yet appearing expressionless because all the character has been zapped from their skin. Do your utmost to find a skilled dermatologist who will go slow at first. Botox and Reloxin wear off—but you don't want to look unnaturally encased in ice until they do.

I often treat patients who need bad work undone. One woman had Botox injected near her eyebrows by someone who was a little heavy-handed. Fast-forward to a few nights later, when she ran into her regular physician at a benefit. He took one look at her face and gasped, "Come see me tomorrow." Her eyelids were sagging so heavily he thought she had myasthenia gravis, a serious and potentially fatal neurological disorder. He didn't think to ask if she'd had a botched Botox job. She didn't think to volunteer that information, because her doctor hadn't bothered to warn her of the small possibility of side effects—one of which was severe eyelid drooping.

So what happened? This terrified woman had an MRI, several CAT scans, paid thousands and thousands of dollars, and had many worried, sleepless nights before her new team of doctors told her she seemed to be fine . . . and the Botox gradually wore off and her eyelids stopped sagging. I convinced her that there was nothing wrong with Botox and her eyelids wouldn't ever droop so severely again—if she were injected properly. I've been seeing her twice a year ever since.

It's also imperative to keep taking good care of your skin and using sun protection after your Botox or Reloxin shots.

Over-the-Counter (OTC) Skin-Care Products

Forehead lines and wrinkles are best treated by Botox or Reloxin. Please see chapter 5 for more information on how to treat regular wrinkles.

That said, an OTC wrinkle relaxer is an ideal Botox support product. The longer you use one, the more potent its effect.

Wrinkle Relaxers

Bliss Crease Police

Caudalie Lifting Serum

DERMAdoctor Immobile Lines Instant Topical Line Relaxer

Dr. Brandt Crease Release

Fredric Brandt, MD

Prescription Topicals

Use a retinoid to keep fine wrinkles at bay.

Injectible Fillers

While Botox and Reloxin are sensational for superficial to medium lines and wrinkles, for volume loss you'd still need a filler. Best would be CosmoDerm or Restylane. Replacing lost volume also helps minimize lines just like Botox and Reloxin do. I often combine fillers with Botox and Reloxin for maximum results.

If your forehead is drooping, fillers such as Juvéderm can be used along with Botox or Reloxin to plump up the area of the eyebrows and above.

Muscle Freezers

For the treatment of the mechanical lines and wrinkles caused by muscle use, Botox and Reloxin rule the forehead!

For uneven eyebrows, realize that most people do have some level of unevenness, and you don't necessarily want to make eyebrows perfectly even. But if you want to even them out, you can use a combination of primarily Botox backed up with a bit of filler.

As for duration, there's no infallible method of predicting how long the results will last. I tell my patients to expect an average of about four months. The more you are injected, the longer the results last, especially when you can break the frowning habit.

Chemical Peels

These would be done on your entire face, not just your forehead.

Lasers

While you can use peels to improve the *texture* of the skin on your forehead, peels and lasers are *not* recommended for lines and wrinkles. Because the lines of the forehead are mostly mechanical in nature, whatever good the peel does will quickly be undone by repetitive use of the muscles. After all, you aren't going to stop smiling, are you?

10-Minute Tips

- Be aware of how much you are inadvertently frowning during the day. Keep a small mirror nearby to remind yourself—and try to break the habit.

- The better you are at managing stress, the less likely you are to furrow your brow.

- During the day, use an OTC anti-oxidant cream and an anti-glycation cream.

- Use a collagen-promoting cream at night. It will help improve skin texture and soften lines.

- Some of my patients like to tape their foreheads at night. They swear it works! If you want to try it, feel free, but it isn't a replacement for wrinkle relaxers or Botox or Reloxin.

10

Eyes

EYES ARE USUALLY the first feature noticed by friends, loved ones, and strangers—who may be quick to judge if you have drooping eyelids, crepey skin texture, dark circles, or profuse wrinkles. As the skin around the eyes has fewer oil glands than the rest of the face, it's more delicate and needs extra attention. Those who've spent a lot of time in the sun or squinting through cigarette smoke are all too aware of how the eye area can show damage more quickly than the cheeks or chin.

No matter what bothers you about your eyes, you will need to use a good eye cream, day and night. These creams work to hydrate and protect the skin, helping to minimize puffiness and dehydrated skin. They should be gentler than regular moisturizers to lessen the possibility of eye irritation, but they also tend to be more occlusive, so use sparingly and never rub. Softly pat them on. If your daytime eye cream doesn't have an SPF, be sure to apply sunscreen afterward, being careful not to get it into your eyes.

If your eyelids are suddenly beginning to droop, or are drooping more noticeably, see a physician or cosmetic surgeon. (You want to rule out the disease myasthenia gravis, which can cause eyelid droop.) In some cases, eyelid droop can become so dramatic that vision, especially peripheral, can be compromised. If that happens, surgical intervention may be needed to remove excess skin. This is not considered a cosmetic procedure, so it may well be reimbursable by insurance.

Another common condition is called *milia*. These are small, round, whitish, benign cysts filled with keratin that appear under the skin, most commonly around the eyes. Sometimes they're triggered by overzealous dermabrasion or a reaction to sunscreen, but most appear with no trigger. They can only be treated by a dermatologist, who will remove them.

1. CREPEY SKIN ON THE EYELIDS AND AROUND THE EYE, AND LOSS OF FIRMNESS

Crepey skin is tough to treat, especially on the thin, vulnerable areas around the eye. However, if you stick to a daily regimen with a good eye cream as well as moisturizers with AHAs, anti-oxidants like vitamin C or vitamin A, and low concentrations of peptides, you should gradually see an improvement in texture. Skin should also become firmer. Discontinue use of any OTC moisturizers if you experience stinging or burning.

Over-the-Counter (OTC) Skin-Care Products

For a list of recommended AHA, anti-oxidant, and peptide treatment creams, refer to page 121 in chapter 5.

Eye Creams

Clinique Repairwear Intensive Eye Cream

Decléor Hydra Floral Deeply Hydrating Eye Contour Gel-Cream

DERMAdoctor Wrinkle Revenge Rescue & Protect Eye Balm

Dr. Brandt Lineless Eye Cream

Dr. Brandt R3P Eye Cream

Kinerase Intensive Eye Cream

Fredric Brandt, MD

Prescription Topicals

Do *not* use any retinoids on the upper-eye area.

For crepey skin underneath the eye, you can try the lowest possible dose and gentlest vehicle for a retinoid, such as Renova. You must use a moisturizer as well as sunscreen, or skin could become very irritated.

Injectible Fillers

Fillers can be used to lift up the eyebrow.

If you have fine little lines in the eyelid, they can be injected with Cosmo-Derm—although you need a dermatologist with extensive experience and a very steady hand. This procedure must be done with extreme care.

If the lower eyelid area is hollow, giving you a tired appearance and dark circles, a filler such as Restylane or CosmoDerm can be used to plump up some of the winkles and improve texture there.

When I inject the Restylane around the eye, I call it the "Restylane pillow" because it provides a pad around the eye, making you look more rested and relaxed. It fills in hollowness and helps reduce puffiness around the eyes, widens the aperture of the eye, and blends in well with any fillers you may have gotten in the cheeks.

Chemical Peels

A superficial peel can help skin texture. It can also be done up to the tarsal plate, which is right at the fold going into the middle of the eyelid. Start with the lowest possible concentration to avoid irritation.

Those brave enough to endure a deep peel will also see an improvement in texture, but the recuperation and pain factors must be considered.

Lasers

Ablative lasers can be used, but this is a tricky procedure, as they may penetrate too deep and could damage the eye itself if wielded by an inexperienced hand.

Other lasers, however, will improve skin texture. Discuss options with your dermatologist.

2. CROW'S-FEET AND WRINKLES

There are two basic treatments for crow's-feet: OTC wrinkle relaxers for short-term results, and Botox and Reloxin, the home-run hitters with long-term results. Crow's-feet are mechanical lines from repeated use (squinting, eye movement) and respond extremely well to muscle freezers. For an extra boost, a filler will intensify the Botox's or Reloxin's effect by plumping up pre-existing hollowness in the area. Peels and lasers can help, but frankly, Botox and Reloxin work so well that I wouldn't spend the time or money doing anything else.

Over-the-Counter (OTC) Skin-Care Products

Wrinkle Relaxers

Bliss Crease Police

Caudalie Lifting Serum

DERMAdoctor Immobile Lines Instant Topical Line Relaxer

Dr. Brandt Crease Release

Injectible Fillers

Fillers designed for fine lines, like collagen or Restylane Fine Lines, will fill in the hollowness in that area prior to Botox or Reloxin, improving results.

It's best to separate the procedures to avoid the bruising that can occur if both are done at the same time. The filler should be injected first.

Muscle Freezers

Botox and Reloxin work wonders for crow's-feet. They can be used to raise the eyebrows and to decrease some of the sagging skin on the upper eyelid. Bear in mind, however, that they tend not to last as long around the eyes as they do in the forehead, as the muscles near the eyes are constantly in use. In this area, these must be injected only by experts, as they can cause double vision if the toxin migrates.

3. DARK CIRCLES

Dark circles under the eyes are caused by either pigmentation, or, more commonly, by blood vessels that appear due to the fragile, thinner, more translucent nature of the skin around the eye. Or by both.

The trick is to differentiate which is causing the dark circles. Anti-pigment agents won't help if the problem is vascular (related to blood vessels) and vice versa.

Over-the-Counter (OTC) Skin-Care Products

If the dark circles are caused by pigmentation, try using a lightener/brightener mixed with your moisturizing eye cream. If there's no improvement after at least six to eight weeks of regular use, the problem may be vascular in nature.

Be sure to try a soothing, anti-inflammatory, anti-oxidant treatment cream, which may help minimize the dark circles as well.

Lighteners/Brighteners

B. Kamins Skin Lightening Treatment

Cellex-C Fade Away Gel

Clarins Bright Plus Total Brightening Serum

Dr. Brandt Laser Lightning Serum

Anti-Oxidant Eye Creams

Dr. Brandt Lineless Eye Cream

Dr. Brandt R3P Eye Cream

Prevage

Physician's Complex C-Plus Anti-Oxidant Serum

SkinMedica Dermal Repair Cream

Injectible Fillers

Restylane can be injected to plump up the skin, which will minimize the appearance of the blood vessels. This does work well, but your dermatologist needs to be very careful, as bruising is a likely (but temporary) result.

Lasers

Certain vascular lasers have been tried on dark circles, but I don't think they're all too successful. If you do have pigment there, you can use certain lasers like the Ruby or the Gemini, which will give some improvement.

4. PUFFINESS AND BAGS UNDER THE EYES

Unfortunately, some people have a genetic predisposition to fatty tissue that happens to land under the eyes, leading to bags and puffiness. Protruding bags worsen as we grow older, as skin weakens and becomes less resilient.

Some of my patients have run right to the cosmetic surgeon to redrape the skin and have the bags removed. Surgery is sometimes extremely successful; other times less so, because when too much fat is removed, the area becomes hollow and you can end up looking even older than you did before the procedure. (Some of my patients who've come for help have wound up resembling cadavers post-surgery—not exactly a youthful look!)

Ironically, puffiness can also occur when you've lost that fat cushion and your collagen and elastin are breaking down, causing surrounding skin to pooch out. It might seem paradoxical, but injecting a filler around the under-eye bag can actually make it seem smaller. Fillers will replace lost volume and disguise or fill in around the hollows or bags of the eye.

Over-the-Counter (OTC) Skin-Care Products

Use a collagen promoter to increase production in the area.

Collagen Promoters/Retinols

Dr. Brandt R3P Eye Cream

NeoStrata Renewing Cream

SkinCeuticals Retinol Complex

SkinMedica Retinol Complex

Injectible Fillers

I tend to use Restylane to improve bags and puffiness and to reduce hollowness.

10-Minute Tips

- Always use an eye cream. Pat it on gently on the orbital bone around the eye and avoid the area close to your lashes. This takes less than a minute!

- Squinting causes wrinkles. Add a UV filter coating to your sunglasses, and choose frames that are larger, rather than on the smallish side, with adequate protection near the corners of your eyes.

- Cool, gel-filled masks or slices of cucumber are instant eye soothers when you're tired or stressed.

- Go to sleep 10 minutes earlier each night—up till the point where you're getting adequate rest. Fatigue shows up immediately in the eye area.

- The smoke from cigarettes is a killer when it comes to eyes.

- For puffiness, decrease your salt intake and try to keep your head slightly elevated when you go to sleep.

- A little bit of caffeine (from one to two cups or coffee) can help decrease puffiness.

- Many of the OTC products sold for under-eye dark circles are *not* treatment creams. They work by refracting light. Make sure you use a *treatment* cream around the eye, preferably one with anti-oxidants.

11

Nose

THE NOSE IS MADE from cartilage, not bone, which has a natural propensity to descend with age. I've had many patients who try to joke, telling me that they're starting to feel like Pinocchio, especially if they have prominent tips. Sometimes they really wonder if they're going crazy—but I hasten to assure them that they're not. Noses really can become longer, while the bones of the skull shrink slightly over time. The result is a larger, drooping nose and an unhappy owner!

Another problem with the nose is a change in skin texture. It's quite common for pores to become enlarged. If that happens, read chapter 8 for suggestions about how to treat them.

Sometimes changes in skin texture and a sort of creeping redness aren't caused by large pores, but by rosacea. An enlargement of the oil glands, which can lead to an enlargement of the nose itself, is one sign of rosacea. Blood vessels on the nose can be treated with vascular lasers, such as the Vbeam and the Aura. For more information about rosacea, read chapter 20.

If you have bumps in your nose, these can only be fixed by surgical intervention (called rhinoplasty). I sometimes treat patients who've been living with the results of botched rhinoplasty years before and are now suffering from indentations or hollows. If that happens, an injectible filler such as Restylane can restore a more even contour to the nose.

Noses need TLC, too, so be sure to keep them hydrated and covered with sunscreen every day.

DROOPING NOSES

Muscle Freezers

A droopy tip responds surprisingly well to Botox and Reloxin, so I suggest you try that before undergoing the pain and expense of surgery. The injection is placed under the tip of the nose and immediately lifts it up.

Make sure your dermatologist has experience doing this procedure.

10-Minute Tips

- Botox is a much quicker fix for a nose droop than cosmetic surgery.

- Always put adequate sunscreen on your nose. It tends to get overlooked (hard as that is to believe).

- Noses are prone to blackheads and whiteheads. These can be treated with a purifying mask. Use it once a week if you have dry or combination skin, and twice a week if you have oily skin.

- Treat the pores on your nose as you would the pores on the rest of your face.

- See a dermatologist if the skin on your nose undergoes any changes.

12

The Fall of the Mid-Face

As we age, the fat deposits (called malar fat pads) inside our cheeks shift and begin to sag and droop. For those in a normal weight range, it seems as though fullness disappears. And those who are very lean can look downright gaunt.

The fall of the mid-face is inevitable, intrinsic, whatever you want to call it—it's responsible for the loss of volume in our faces. Dealing with this problem is more complicated than a mere filling in of lines, which can actually produce a kind of lumpen heaviness in the area and is hardly an optimal result. In addition, one of the biggest fallacies about how to treat the fall of the mid-face comes from overzealous cosmetic surgeons and gullible women who consult them. Patients often think that face-lifts are the only treatment that can improve the naso-labial fold, or the smile lines between the nose and the lips. I hasten to tell my patients that this simply isn't true.

Face-lifts can be great for contouring the jawline and removing excess skin there. During the lift, there will be some pulling up of the cheeks, but to my mind that's not what really constitutes a youthful face. A youthful face has a full, curving, rounded contour. Once this contour is gone, say hello to the naso-labial fold.

Nearly all of my patients think that their naso-labial fold is an isolated sign of aging. But the naso-labial fold isn't the problem—it's the *symptom*. The cause of the problem is the loss of volume and falling malar fat pads.

This is why I never like to treat the naso-labial fold on its own. The falling malar fat pads don't just affect the cheeks—they can push down and create the marionette lines running between the lip and the chin, and leave either puffiness or hollowness under the eyes as well as wrinkles around it. Again, this is caused by a volume loss of fat and the reduction of collagen around the eyes.

By replacing lost volume, you instantly pick up not only the entire mid-face area—rounding out the cheeks and diminishing the naso-labial fold—but you'll also smooth out the lines running down from the lips and the hollowness or puffiness around the eyes.

By treating the mid-face, you can once again have a youthful contour. It's like stuffing a sofa. If you lose the stuffing, everything starts sagging and falling. Fill it back in, and the sofa becomes nice and plump, and smooth, again.

When a patient brings in their high school yearbook picture, I can compare that little snapshot with how they look today. This concept was perfectly proven one day, when Samantha Saunders, who was fifty-five, came in with her daughter, Roxanne, who was twenty-four. Samantha was not happy with her naso-labial fold, and Roxanne needed help with some complexion problems. It was a great tool to have Roxanne there, because she had similar facial characteristics to her mother's. And looking at her daughter was like having a live mirror held up to Samantha's face when she was younger.

"Look at your daughter's cheeks," I told Samantha. "If you want to lift up your cheek like your daughter's, this will take care of ninety percent of your naso-labial fold problem, and also soften the eye area and give you back the volume that you've been losing over time. Then you'll have the youthful characteristics of a beautiful face, with lovely round cheeks."

"Like Ingrid Bergman's," Samantha said.

"Oh, Mom," said Roxanne. "You mean like Angelina Jolie, or Charlize Theron."

"Like all three," I said.

"Just don't make me look like Humphrey Bogart," Samantha said with a laugh.

"Don't worry," I told her. "I won't."

A few words of caution:

- Be very wary of any dermatologist or plastic surgeon who tells you that one filler fits all for treatment of the mid-face. It doesn't. I almost always mix and match, concocting a unique cocktail of fillers, to inject in this area. When adding volume, I'm injecting material into the mid to deeper dermis, where the defect is. If you have wrinkles, however, the defect is in the upper portion of the dermis, so you need a much finer material to do the trick. The higher up in the dermis, the more superficial the wrinkle, and the finer the material is. It is simply not possible to use the same material to replace lost volume as you would to fill in fine lines. No one substance can take care of everything at once.

- Nor should you come to see me, or any other cosmetic dermatologist, to deal with volume loss until you're over thirty. Except for a handful of extreme cases, volume loss does not truly begin until the mid-thirties or so. I advise women in their twenties (and, I hate to say, even some teenagers) that volume loss is not an issue for them now. Protecting their skin from the sun should be their number one priority. They should plan on coming back to see me in another ten years or so, and we'll deal with the issue then, if need be.

- Botox and Reloxin are *never* recommended for the cheek area. They can't be used to smooth the naso-labial fold, or to add volume to the cheeks. Walk right out the door if anyone says they are! Botox and Reloxin work by temporarily blocking the nerve impulses that control muscle movement, and would restrict your ability to contract your facial muscles. No movement means no wrinkles. But paralyzing muscles in the cheek area will affect how you move your mouth. Not a good thing!

- Although cosmetic surgeons may say otherwise, I almost never recommend cheek implants. They often look fake, they can feel terrible, the surgery is painful and can leave scars, and fillers are so much simpler. Besides, it's so much easier to undo a filler, which will gradually disappear, than it is to undo a botched implant.

180

1. CHEEK WRINKLES

For fine wrinkles on the cheeks, alpha hydroxy acids (AHAs) are most commonly used. In addition, you can choose an OTC cream containing retinol or peptides, both of which help stimulate collagen production, which can improve the quality and texture of your skin. Wrinkle relaxers and skin smoothers will also help.

See your dermatologist for prescription retinoids and other treatments, such as peels and laser resurfacing.

For detailed information about wrinkles, see chapter 5.

2. VOLUME LOSS

Reestablishing volume in the mid-face makes my patients look younger than just about any other cosmetic dermatologist procedure. It's one of the easiest and most gratifying things I can do. I just love tackling the fall of the mid-face! To me, it's like working on a living sculpture.

Over-the-Counter (OTC) Skin-Care Products

Never believe any claims that an OTC cream can mimic the effects of an injectible filler. It's physiologically *impossible*. It's like comparing apples and oranges; one will never be the other.

That said, it is possible to improve *firmness* and tone with OTC skin-tightening products. These products do improve the skin's elasticity of the skin and help prevent its sagging.

Skin Tighteners

Caudalie Lifting Serum

Clinique Anti-Gravity Firming Lift Cream

Dr. Brandt Contour Effect

Dr. Brandt Laser Tight

Juvena Firming Performance

Lancôme Rénergie Microlift Flash Lifting

Intense Pulsed Light, GentleWaves LED, Photodynamic Therapy, Coblation, Thermage, and Titan

The Titan is quite good for tightening skin in this area, so it can work well as an adjunct procedure when fillers have been used.

Injectible Fillers

Fillers are without question the best and quickest way to replace lost volume in the mid-face.

Many of my patients are surprised when I tell them that. When they do, I tell them that the biggest misconceptions about filler substances is that they're only good to fix lines and wrinkles, or that if you use fillers to replace lost volume, you'll end up with a big, fat, round face! Of course, if an untrained or unskilled hand wields the needle, you may well end up with chipmunk cheeks—but if the right filler is used, in the right places, it can literally take years off your face, in an instant.

Your dermatologist should use a mixture of collagen and hyaluronic acid fillers, and perhaps polylactic acid (Sculptra) for this area. Fat transfer can also be used. Synthetics such as ArteFill and silicone may be injected in certain cases, as long as you're aware of the risks.

3. CHEEK DROOPING:
THE NASO-LABIAL FOLD

Jasmine was sitting in one of my examination rooms, swinging her legs and reading *Allure* magazine. She greeted me enthusiastically as I scanned her new patient information form, then asked what I could do to help.

"It's these lines next to my nose, Doc," she said, running her fingers down from the side of her nostrils to her lips. "They're so big. They're really bugging me. I just hate them. Can you fix them, like, now?"

I carefully examined Jasmine's skin, and when I gently told her that her lines weren't actually big enough to fix—that they were, in fact, practically nonexistent—her face fell.

"Really?" she cried. "Are you sure? They're just so awful!"

Jasmine was nineteen years old.

I see many young women like Jasmine, who have an exaggerated fear of the lines near their nose, especially if they think it's going to make them instantly turn into their mother. But rare indeed is the patient who needs these lines fixed before her mid-thirties. Small naso-labial fold lines are perfectly normal, in children, teens, and young women. Trying to "fix" them prematurely actually *adds* years to a face.

So I told Jasmine that she'd have lots of time to do procedures when she was older, but in the meantime, she should stop smoking (I could smell it on her breath) and use a good broad-spectrum sunscreen to protect her skin. That would keep her skin in much better shape than anything I could do for her in the foreseeable future.

As I said earlier in this chapter, nearly all of my patients think that their naso-labial fold is the cause of their falling mid-face. Again, the naso-labial fold isn't the problem—it's the *symptom*. The cause of the problem is the loss of volume and falling fat pads. It's not enough just to add a filler to the fold itself. That's like putting a Band-Aid on a gaping wound; it's not strong enough to fix the problem. What *will* fix the problem is to add volume to the cheek area in the form of a filler substance first and then tackle the fold. That lifts the cheek area up and away from the naso-labial fold, so less filler will be needed in the fold itself.

I'd be tremendously skeptical of any physician who only recommends a filler for a deep naso-labial fold itself. Make sure your entire mid-face area will be treated to improve this problem.

Some plastic surgeons have used Gore-Tex or Ultra Soft Form implants, which are permanent, synthetic substances, to fill in the naso-labial fold, but I do not recommend them. They can look decidedly lumpen and unnatural.

Injectible Fillers

Discuss all the options with your dermatologist, who should be treating you with a combination of collagen, hyaluronic acids, polylactic acid, and your own harvested fat. As ever, be informed about permanent fillers (ArteFill and silicone) prior to their use.

10-Minute Tips

- I sound like a broken record already, but keep your mid-face protected from the sun.

- Smoke from cigarettes affects this part of the face, too.

- Using an OTC lifting product can help improve the appearance of lines and wrinkles on the cheeks.

13

Lips

I nearly keeled over the first time I heard that phrase, used with a snicker by one of my patients in Miami. She opened the latest issue of one of the tabloids and pointed to a lurid color photograph of the abnormally puffy lips of a Hollywood superstar.

"Yep," said my patient. "She's got a trout pout alright. Isn't it awful? It's just so *fake*. Just like when Goldie Hawn had it done in *The First Wives Club*."

In that case, I had to agree that whoever had injected the superstar had indeed gone too far—at least to my trained eye. But who's to say if the physician was to blame, or if the superstar had demanded more, more, and then some more?

Lips naturally thin and shrink with age. And, of course, with sun damage they get worse. The primary solution at our disposal is injectible filler.

The ease with which lips can be injected with these fillers, and the lovely, natural, albeit unusually large shape of Angelina Jolie's lips have led to a near-epidemic of grossly inflated puckers. Not only are these lips obviously filled, but the current esthetic is to create lips that are disproportionately large for their owners' faces.

To me, this is akin to anorexia, or body dysmorphic disorder, where people have a distorted view of how they truly look. Just as some body builders pumped up full of steroids get bigger and bigger yet can't stop pumping, some women who fill up their lips don't think they're actually that big anymore. With patients like that, I try to reestablish the boundaries and bring them down to reality. Sometimes I succeed. Sometimes I don't. Unfortunately, there's always a physician somewhere who will be all too happy to give patients whatever they want.

An ethical and compassionate dermatologist will do his or her utmost to create the desired lip—within reason. I always ask my patients exactly what kind of lip shape or size they're thinking about. Some of them will even bring an ad with a model, or a photograph of a celebrity, and I often have to disappoint them when I gently explain that there's only so much I can and will do to alter the natural line of their lips. Someone with naturally thin lips will look freakish if she suddenly inflates them to Angelina's proportions.

What's crucial for me is to assess the size of the patient's face; the bigger the face, the bigger the lips can be. Whatever the size, they need to be nicely shaped, with even borders. I use a 3:2 ratio—the bottom lip should be a little bit bigger than the top lip. Sometimes my patients want a much larger top lip, but I find that if the top lip is bigger than the bottom, there's no support for it, and it hangs over the mouth. The most important factor as you age is to raise up the corners of the lip. That often involves shortening the upper lip and lengthening the lower lip. Plus you want to decrease the distance from the mouth to the nose, which also increases with age.

All of these factors should be taken into consideration and discussed prior to any injections. You certainly don't want the dreaded trout pout to be the first thing anyone will notice about you!

Fortunately, most of my patients are merely hoping to once more have the lip volume they had a decade before, but with a little more definition. They want subtle enhancement. Restoring that volume is not complicated and is an extremely gratifying procedure.

Fredric Brandt, MD

1. THINNING LIPS

Over-the-Counter (OTC) Skin-Care Products

Topical lip plumpers have exploded in popularity. A few years ago there were only a handful on the market, and now there are dozens. I wish I could say I wholeheartedly endorse these plumpers, but I can't. Frankly, I think many of them are truly dreadful, as they work in a negative way—by causing irritation. The active ingredient that does this is most likely from the Capsicum family. You know—hot red cayenne pepper. Or the irritation can be caused by caffeine, menthol, or cinnamon oil. Put on a lip plumper with any of those ingredients, and they can sting and burn until you rush into the bathroom to wash them off.

Injectible Fillers

I think that the hyaluronic acids are the stars when it comes to filling and plumping up the lips. I most often use Restylane or Juvéderm, with perhaps some CosmoPlast (collagen) on the border of the lip. I've found that Restylane gives you a nice soft lip, and it holds really well, up to six months. The more frequently you're injected, the longer it seems to last. And as Restylane can be dissolved, if your dermatologist was heavy-handed, or you're not crazy about your new lips, they can be undone.

Silicone can be used in micro-droplets to gradually enlarge the lips, but this must be done with extreme care, as it's a permanent substance. Sculptra and ArteFill are not recommended for use in the lips.

2. WRINKLES ON THE LIPS

Believe it or not, lips get more than merely chapped. They do wrinkle, especially the lower lip. It's as important to exfoliate the lips as it is to exfoliate the skin, and to work on increasing collagen production in the lips to help the little lines and wrinkles.

Keep lips hydrated at all times with moisturizing lip balms. Look for those with natural ingredients and as little fragrance and dye as possible, and apply them often. Hydrated lips will always look plumper than dry ones. Bear in mind that lip balms with sunscreen do protect lips from the sun but can be irritating.

Over-the-Counter (OTC) Skin-Care Products

Lip Balms

Alba Organics Lip Balm

BeesWork Organic Lip Balm

Benefit Lipscription

Clarins Extra-Firming Age-Control Lip + Contour Care

Fresh Sugar Lip Balm

GoSmile SmileCeuticals Lip Balm

NARS Lip Therapy

3. WRINKLES AROUND THE LIPS

Wrinkles on the skin around the upper lip can become very tough to treat. They're formed by pursing action over the years. Some of my patients naturally purse their lips as they talk; others like to drink through straws, which doesn't help either. The other likely culprit is smoking. Smokers, as you know by now, also tend to wrinkle more easily anyway, and their wrinkles are more difficult to eradicate.

If you do have a tendency to purse your lips, try to become more aware of the habit so you can put an end to it. Less pursing will lead to increased longevity if you have any injected fillers in the area.

Some patients have come to see me with upper-lip wrinkles so deep they won't go away by stretching the skin. For them, fillers can help only so much. Their only other alternative is a deep peel, which can be problematic.

Bottom line: Don't let lip wrinkles get bad. Stop smoking, stay out of the sun, try not to purse, and keep the area hydrated.

Over-the-Counter (OTC) Skin-Care Products

Refer to the information on wrinkles in chapter 5. Use your choice of OTC AHAs, anti-oxidants, or peptide creams. Home microdermabrasion and home peels with glycolic acid will have a slight effect, depending on the severity of the wrinkles.

Prescription Topicals

A retinoid will help with superficial wrinkles.

Mechanical Exfoliation

A course of microdermabrasion is definitely recommended.

Injectible Fillers

For mild to moderate wrinkles, fillers such as CosmoDerm, Zyderm, and Resty-lane Fine Lines can be used. Micro-droplets of silicone can also be injected.

Muscle Freezers

It's a tricky procedure, but Botox or Reloxin can be used in very low concentrations (called mild relaxation) to help soften some of the superficial wrinkles. They won't help deep wrinkles.

Botox and Reloxin can also be used in combination with injectible fillers, especially for those who tend to purse a lot. Be sure your dermatologist knows the exact dosage and is experienced in injecting these substances so close to the mouth.

Chemical Peels

Superficial and moderate peels can help superficial to moderate wrinkles; deep wrinkles necessitate deeper peels, which have a serious pain factor and recuperation.

One of the big problems with upper-lip wrinkles is that they're often worse than the wrinkles on the rest of the face, but the area can't be treated on its own with a deep peel. (You need to treat the whole upper lip, lower lip, and chin.) Deep CO_2 peels can de-pigment the area, and you'd need to wear makeup all the time to even out your skin tone. And as a deep phenol peel is a drastic procedure, deciding to undergo one is a difficult decision to make.

Lasers

For some reason, non-ablative lasers as well as Fraxel don't work as well on upper-lip wrinkles as they do on the face. The only alternative is a CO_2 laser, but as with peels, it should only be done if the whole face is treated, with a heavier dose given to the upper-lip area. Again, this is a procedure that can work, but involves much pain and recuperation.

10-Minute Tips

- Try not to purse your lips.

- Avoid using straws, as this automatically causes a pursing action.

- No sucking on cigarettes!

- Keep lip balm handy—at your desk, in your handbag, near the door, by your bed.

- Lip plumpers usually work through irritation. Buyer beware!

- You don't need to exfoliate your lips—unlike the skin on your face, there's no stratum corneum, the topmost layer of dead skin cells, so there's no reason to slough this layer off.

- Stay away from tartar control toothpaste if you develop irritation around your lips.

- Your lower lip gets more sun exposure than the top, so it needs more sun protection.

14

Chin

DON'T THINK YOU'RE GOING CRAZY if you wonder why your lower face seems to be going south as you age. Chins *do* lengthen. A charming picture, right?

The biggest concern in the chin area is what's called the oral commissures, or the marionette lines, running from the sides of the lips and then down the chin. They're caused by a few factors: a loss of the support tissue such as fat and collagen in the chin; dental problems, such as gum erosion and bone loss due to teeth grinding; or the activity of the *depressor anguli oris muscle* of the mouth, which pulls everything down, making your face look sad, tired, or unhappy—even when you're not. As a result, it's important to see someone who can treat this area with some kind of injectible filler to build up the support tissue in the chin.

Another chin problem is dimpling due to volume loss.

Often, when the cheek area is treated, it helps pick up the marionette lines as well.

CHIN (MARIONETTE) LINES AND DIMPLING

Over-the-Counter (OTC) Skin-Care Products

Most OTC products are not capable of treating the marionette lines, as they are deep grooves. The best choice would be any of the creams that stimulate collagen production, as well as wrinkle relaxers. Refer to pages 119–22 in chapter 5 for more information.

Injectible Fillers

Any of the injectible fillers with a moderate density, such as Restylane or Juvéderm, can be used to de-groove the marionette lines and fill in dimples. Results are quickly visible.

Muscle Freezers

Another treatment for marionette lines is to relax the muscles that pull down the corners of the mouth, and this can be done with Botox or Reloxin. Injections in the platysmal muscles of the neck also help lift the chin.

Botox or Reloxin can also be injected into the mentalis muscle of the chin, which relaxes the contraction that causes a lot of the dimpling. This can be combined with a filler if the dimpling is severe.

As ever, a very deft hand is needed with the chin, because the result could be an asymmetrical smile, or, in the worst-case scenario, there could be a temporary paralysis of some of the muscles needed to move the mouth. This could be devastating to anyone who's, for example, a singer, musician, teacher, or public speaker, who needs to use these muscles in order to work.

If you're considering Botox or Reloxin, realize that good results on the lower face are definitely more dependent on doctor technique than the upper face is, so proceed accordingly!

10-Minute Tips

- Be aware of how you smile. I see many of my patients inadvertently pulling down the corners of their mouths when they smile. Over time, this will definitely contribute to the formation of marionette lines. Ask a friend to tell you when you're doing it, or keep a hand mirror handy, so you can see how you move your mouth, and try to correct it.

- Tooth grinding can affect your chin!

- Keep your gums healthy and never miss a dentist's appointment. The healthier your gums, the less likely you are to suffer bone loss—which contributes to the changes in the shape of your chin (and not for the better).

15

Jawline

BOTOX AND RELOXIN are modern marvels that have erased forehead wrinkles from millions of happy people. And they also have another fabulous effect on the jawline. In fact, they can be so effective at lifting drooping jowls and improving the jawline that I call what they can do the Botox and Reloxin Face-lifts. Actually, it's really a neck-lift, as, ironically, the injections are not placed in the jawline itself, but in the cords (platysmal bands) of the neck. This takes the downward pull away and gives a big boost to the entire area resting above them. I'm extremely proud of this procedure, as it's one I developed myself and perfected over the years.

Don't get me wrong—face-lifts can work wonders for those who have a large amount of sagging in the face and neck caused by the inevitable loss of volume due to less fat and collagen as well as deteriorating collagen and elastin. But for many who aren't quite yet as droopy, an injectible face-lift is a far less costly and invasive treatment for jowls, with no downtime. It's effective for those who've never had a face-lift as well as those who've already had one (or more), yet are beginning to sag again due to the inevitability of gravity. And it works!

JOWLS AND DROOPING JAWLINE

Over-the-Counter (OTC) Skin-Care Products

OTC tighteners will help increase the elasticity of the skin by improving the quality and quantity of collagen.

Skin Tighteners/Collagen Promoters

Caudalie Lifting Serum

Clinique Anti-Gravity Firming Lift Cream

Dr. Brandt Contour Effect

Dr. Brandt Laser Tight

Juvena Firming Performance

Lancôme Rénergie Microlift Flash Lifting

Intense Pulsed Light, GentleWaves LED, Photodynamic Therapy, Coblation, Thermage, and Titan

The Titan can give sensational results, as it tightens and lifts the jawline. Other dermatologists recommend Thermage, but I prefer the Titan, as it's much less painful and gives, in my opinion, more predictable results.

Injectible Fillers

Any of the mid to deep fillers—Sculptra, Restylane, or Juvéderm—will help restore the contour of the jawline. Silicone may be recommended, but with the usual cautions.

Muscle Freezers

The Botox neck-lift will definitely elevate the jawline and reduce jowls.

10-Minute Tips

- Try the least invasive procedure first. You may not need a face-lift even if your friends tell you that you do!

- Your jawline needs the same amount of treatment creams and sun protection as the rest of your face. Be sure to apply products evenly.

16

Neck

THE NECK OFTEN GIVES AWAY a woman's age. The skin there is extremely delicate, with fewer of the oil glands that help facial skin heal and repair itself, so it's much more prone to damage and scarring than the face. It can be neglected when moisturizers and anti-aging creams and sunscreen are slathered carefully each day elsewhere on the face and body. As a result, the skin on the neck can become wrinkled, loose, riddled with hyperpigmentation spots or broken blood vessels, and develop a crepey texture. In addition, the cords (platysmal bands) can become more prominent, giving a strained look.

Taking care of your neck (and don't forget the décolleté) is as important as taking care of your face. Always apply sunscreen and moisturizers to the neck and décolleté whenever you apply them to your face.

Over-the-Counter (OTC) Skin-Care Products

Neck creams aren't luxury products or designed to trick consumers into thinking they need to buy yet another skin-care cream. They're designed to treat the loss of elasticity and decreased collagen production, and are usually gentler and slightly more occlusive than face creams.

For crepey texture, use any of the AHA, anti-oxidant, retinol, or peptide creams. See pages 119–22 in chapter 5 for more information.

For hyperpigmentation spots, see pages 139–41 and 144 in chapter 6.

Neck Creams

Clarins Advanced Extra-Firming Neck Cream

Dr. Brandt V-Zone Neck Cream

Dr. Brandt Crease Release

Dr. Brandt Laser Tight

Z. Bigatti Re-Storation Swan Firming Neck Treatment

Prescription Topicals

Retinoids will reduce wrinkles and crepey texture. Renova is the most gentle, so I recommend it for the tender skin of the neck.

Intense Pulsed Light, GentleWaves LED, Photodynamic Light Therapy, Coblation, Thermage, and Titan

IPL can work to improve sun damage and superficial wrinkles. GentleWaves is also a good treatment, as it's very gentle for this area and will help skin texture. The Titan or Thermage can be also used to tighten the skin and diminish wrinkles.

Injectible Fillers

Use only superficial fillers like CosmoDerm or Restylane Fine Lines. These will improve superficial wrinkles.

Muscle Freezers

Botox or Reloxin injected into the neck will diminish the downward pull on the cords (platysmal bands) and horizontal lines due to muscle hypertrophy, and eliminate wrinkling in the neck and décolleté.

Chemical Peels

Only the most superficial peels can be used on the neck, as it doesn't heal as well as the face.

Lasers

Non-ablative lasers and Fraxel will improve crepey texture.

Hyperpigmentation spots are treated with pigment lasers, either the Q-switch ruby, Q-switch alexandrite, Q-switch Nd:YAG, or Aura.

Dilated, broken blood vessels, a condition called *poikiloderma*, are treated with one of the vascular lasers that target red pigment. Use the VersaPulse, Aura, or Vbeam vascular laser.

10-Minute Tips

- Don't forget to moisturize your neck.

- If you don't have a special neck cream, use a regular moisturizer.

- Apply sunscreen evenly on the front and back of your neck.

- See a dermatologist as soon as you notice textural changes, like crepeyness. The earlier it's treated, the better.

- When exercising, try not to tighten your neck muscles too much. Avoid straining!

17

Ears

IF THE NECK IS NEGLECTED, pity the ears! How often do you put sunscreen on them? Every day? Or just when you're on vacation at a beach resort? I rest my case.

Ears are made of cartilage, a spongy substance that has no bone in it. Gravity does its dirty work on them, too, so as years go by, ears become thinner and droop down. Not only do collagen and elastin deteriorate, but the constant pulling due to the weight of earrings takes its toll. When earlobes elongate, the results can be alarming—in extreme cases, they can reach the chin level (or lower!).

Many of my patients are surprised when I tell them that ears can be plumped up with fillers. Obviously, the sooner you have your ears treated, the less they will droop. Try to stay away from heavy earrings or wear them as little as possible during the day.

And don't forget to apply sunscreen to your ears whenever you're applying it to your face.

Over-the-Counter (OTC) Skin-Care Products

Any OTC product for wrinkling can be used on the ears. Refer to pages 119–22 in chapter 5 for more information.

Injectible Fillers

Many of my patients erroneously believe that drooping earlobes can only be fixed by surgery that will cut away excess skin, but fillers can do the trick. Adding volume to drooping earlobes plumps them up, actually making them smaller as well as lifted back up. I usually use either collagen or Restylane, or a combination of both.

Chemical Peels

Superficial peels will improve texture and tone. Stay away from any of the more intense peels.

Lasers

Non-ablative lasers can firm ears and remove some of the superficial lines.

10-Minute Tips

- Apply moisturizer to ears just as you would your face.

- Ditto the sunscreen!

- Try to avoid regular use of heavy earrings. If you love them, try to take them off for extended periods to give your earlobes a rest.

- Don't tug on earlobes.

18

Hands

GRAY ROOTS CAN BE DYED; faces can be plumped with fillers and treated with lasers to give them back a lovely, youthful fullness and radiance; but until very recently, hands were an immediate giveaway of age. Their thin, delicate skin, physiological structure, and constant motion lead to the hands showing the effects of age years before the rest of the body.

The primary culprit is, as ever, the sun. Hands are almost constantly exposed to UV radiation, and since we use them so much, sunscreen rubs off quickly. (Of course, this is assuming that sunscreen is even applied in the first place.)

The damage appears as hyperpigmentation spots, wrinkling, loss of elasticity, textural changes, volume loss, and prominent, ropy veins. Much of these changes in texture and pigmentation can be prevented by the simple, regular use of a high SPF sunscreen. I can always tell who plays golf, since one hand (the gloved one, not surprisingly!) looks much better than the other. And many of my patients are surprised when I examine their hands and tell them to wear driving gloves—but not the ones with the little holes in them. It's pretty amazing how much UV radiation passes through the windshield of a car to bombard the hands over the years.

Hand creams with SPF are a must during the day, but you can also use your preferred skin-care products on your hands, too. Just be gentle, as the skin on the hands is fragile.

1. HAND WRINKLES AND CREPEY TEXTURE

Over-the-Counter (OTC) Skin-Care Products

Rough or crepey texture or loss of firmness responds well to OTC treatment. In addition to using hand cream regularly, you can use anti-oxidant, retinol, or peptide creams on your hands. Refer to pages 119–22 in chapter 5 for more information about wrinkle products.

Hand Creams

B. Kamins Maple Treatment Hand Cream SPF 20

Dr. Brandt Hand Cream

Z. Bigatti Enhance Hand and Nail Cream

Prescription Topicals

Retinoids will remove fine wrinkles. Best would be Renova, as skin on the hands may be more sensitive to stronger formulations. Sunscreen is an absolute must with any retinoid.

Chemical Peels

The most superficial peels, with TCA, glycolic, or salicylic acid, will improve texture and remove light wrinkles.

Fredric Brandt, MD

2. HAND HYPERPIGMENTATION

For more information about hyperpigmentation, see chapter 6. OTC lighteners/brighteners can be used on the hands, but you must stick to the regimen to see results.

Over-the-Counter (OTC) Skin-Care Products

Lighteners/Brighteners

B. Kamins Skin Lightening Treatment

Cellex-C Fade Away Gel

Clarins Bright Plus Total Brightening Serum

Dr. Brandt Laser Lightning Serum

MD Formulations Vit-A-Plus Illuminating Creme SPF 15

Intense Pulsed Light, GentleWaves LED, Photodynamic Therapy, Coblation, Thermage, and Titan

IPL and GentleWaves can be used on the hands, but I think that the most potent power of the lasers gives better results.

Lasers

The pigment lasers are specifically designed to target individual brown spots. Best for the hands are the Q-switched ruby, the Q-switched alexandrite, or the Q-switched Nd:YAG laser. To avoid the risk of more hyperpigmentation or hypopigmentation (white spots) after treatment, you must use sunscreen while the skin is healing.

3. HAND VOLUME LOSS AND VEINS

Injectible Fillers

Volume loss in the hands—which can make them look slightly cadaverous—can be treated with Restylane, which that works quite nicely. Juvéderm has excellent results as well, and is now FDA-approved. You may also try fat transfer. I wouldn't recommend Sculptra; as the skin is so thin, you don't want to see lumps and bumps after the injections. I always have my patients sit on their hands after the treatment; this helps compress the filler and gives a more pleasing result.

There are some who would endure surgery to remove prominent veins on their hands, but it's not a procedure I would care to endorse. I suggest you try a filler first, because when skin is plumped up, the veins should automatically be reduced in appearance.

10-Minute Tips

- Hands need pampering. Always coat with sunscreen and reapply often.

- Keep small bottles of hand cream at your desk and by your bed.

- If you've forgotten the hand cream, use a regular facial product. Any with retinol, to increase collagen production, are a good idea.

- For extra hydration, apply a thick layer of a moisturizing cream, then slip on thin cotton gloves before you go to bed.

- Avoid drying nail products, such as polish removers with acetone. Keep cuticles hydrated and never cut them.

- Hands benefit from microdermabrasion and peels too. Just be gentle, as the skin is much thinner and more sensitive than that on the face.

- Wear gloves while driving. Leather driving gloves have a good grip on the steering wheel, but the little holes let in the sun. Try to find thin leather that won't heat up your hands and has a good grip—but with no perforations!

- Hand massage is a great idea to reduce stress and strain, and gives the hands an extra dose of a hydrating cream or massage oil.

19

Hair Loss on the Scalp and Hair Growth on the Face

BETTY LEWIS, AGE FIFTY-TWO, sat on the examining table, brushing her shimmering golden hair back, her eyes brimming with tears. "I'm so embarrassed," she finally whispered. "It's my hair."

I looked at Betty's hair, which was long and thick. Then I looked closer and realized she was wearing a wig, one of the most incredibly lifelike I'd ever seen.

"May I see?" I asked.

She nodded, then whipped off her wig. Her own hair had been cropped short, but I could still see that she had lost much of it, in the classic female pattern of an overall thinning on the top of the head.

"Hair loss is incredibly common in women, you know," I told her. "Between thirty to forty percent of all women over thirty have some hair loss and thinning. So you're not alone."

"But I feel so alone," she said, crying in earnest. "It's just so embarrassing. I don't want anyone to see me."

The hair follicle is a little factory where the hair and its coloring are produced. Normally, 90 percent of hair is in different stages of growth, so no hair loss is evident then. The remaining 10 percent is resting.

When the little factories stop working, hair loss becomes evident. This is

MINUTES/10 YEARS

214 incredibly common condition in women, but talking about it isn't. Worse, it can provoke deep shame and mortification. Fortunately, hair loss can be treated, sometimes with good results. At the very least, even if no new hair growth occurs, the continuing loss of more hair can be halted.

I always recommend that you see your doctor if there's any hair loss. There are different kinds of hair loss, with different treatment regimens. Sometimes hair loss is caused by something as simple as the wrong kind of hairstyle, as tight braids or twists can create traction hair loss. Another form of hair loss, *alopecia areata,* is an auto-immune disorder where hair tends to be lost in a specific area only, usually in circular shapes. I need to rule out that there are no underlying medical conditions, such as thyroid disease, iron deficiency, polycystic ovarian syndrome, or any other medical problems. This is done with blood tests. If it turns out you do have a treatable condition, hair loss will usually stop once the condition improves with the proper medication.

If the scalp and body are healthy, I'll check to see if you have diffuse hair loss, which is often precipitated by a stressful event, surgery, or pregnancy. I'll examine whatever medications and/or supplements you might be taking, as some, like birth control pills and DHEA, can cause hair loss. This hair loss almost always reverses itself when the cause is discovered.

If the hair is thinning in the frontal areas, especially the front of the scalp, there's usually a family history of hair loss or balding. This kind of hair loss is caused by heredity, or your genetic potential; or by a predisposition, which can be caused by certain medical conditions. Most women tend to notice hair loss when they enter perimenopause and/or menopause, when hormones are shifting and menstrual cycles become irregular, along with a host of other symptoms. Female *androgenetic alopecia (AGA),* the most common type of hair loss, is predominantly caused by hormonal shifts or as a side effect of certain medications. As women age, the feminizing hormones (estrogen and progesterone) naturally decline, allowing the masculinizing hormones, or androgens (most notably testosterone), to become elevated. The good news is that prescription anti-androgens will bring the dominating hormones more closely into balance.

And there's another potential cause of hair loss: excessive weight and consumption of sugar. (Remember chapter 2?) Studies have supported the hypothesis that women with some markers of insulin resistance have a significantly higher risk for AGA. The exact link hasn't been proven yet, but anyone at risk for developing type 2 diabetes should be aware that hair loss can accompany weight gain. Often, the androgens decrease as soon as weight is lost. So not only can sugar make you look old, it may cause your hair to fall out, too.

If you are experiencing hair loss, particularly if it comes on suddenly or in large patches, it is imperative to see a physician. I often see a quartet of interconnected conditions—seborrheic dermatitis (mistakenly thought of as plain old dandruff), which is inflammation; hair loss; adult acne; and hair growth on the face—in many of my patients. So don't despair. Instead, see a dermatologist. You *can* be helped!

HAIR LOSS

Over-the-Counter (OTC) Skin-Care Products

Many regular shampoos or tonics that claim to stimulate hair growth just don't work. You'll need to look for specific ingredients that have been proven to lessen hair loss.

Anti-inflammatory and anti-fungal shampoos seem to have anti-androgenic properties. I recommend ketoconazole, sold as Nizoral 1 percent or 2 percent shampoo; and 1 percent pyrithione zinc, sold as Head and Shoulders and Denorex; and DCL Zoma shampoo medicated formula 1.9 percent. You'll usually need to use these shampoos for at least four months before seeing results.

Zinc taken orally also seems to help with hair loss. This is because zinc is an essential component of around two hundred enzymes that are involved in a range of cellular processes, including having an anti-androgenic effect. Take 100 mg each day.

Minoxidil, the chemical name for Rogaine, is available in a 2 percent or 5 percent strength topical solution or as Rogaine Foam OTC. It's applied directly to the scalp. I think the OTC 5 percent solution, originally designed for men, works better for women. These products must absolutely not be used during pregnancy, so consult your doctor prior to any use.

Prescription Medications

Anti-androgen medications come in many different forms. You need to work closely with your dermatologist and gynecologist to find out which one is the best for you. Some are toxic to developing fetuses and must never be used during preg-

---

A HAIRDRESSER'S ADVICE FOR THINNING HAIR

I asked Garren, a well-known hairstylist in Manhattan, for tips about how best to work with thinning hair—something that hairstylists see as regularly as dermatologists do.

- Go to a few consultations with great hairstylists. Although it can be hard to talk about at first, rest assured that they've seen it on many other women and will do their utmost to help. If you find that your concerns are being dismissed, keep looking for a stylist who understands the problem and wants to work with you.

- A skilled stylist can shape hair to disguise some of the hair loss.

- Washing your hair often does not contribute to hair loss, but women who are obsessed with squeaky-clean hair can dry out their scalp with unnecessary shampooing. Use shampoos and conditioners with all-natural ingredients that won't irritate your scalp. Some are designed to add volume, and they can give a temporary thickening effect.

- Don't use too much or too many styling products, as it will show the loss even more.

- Coloring or adding a color rinse to hair automatically plumps up the hair shaft and enriches the volume. I can attest to this personally, thanks to my colorist Kyle White at Oscar Blandi Salon.

- Hair extensions are a possibility, but only if done by a skilled stylist and in a way that they won't pull and increase breakage.

nancy, so always discuss potential pregnancy plans prior to starting any regimen. Most of the anti-androgens take at least four to six months to begin working.

Some of the most commonly prescribed anti-androgens are: finasteride, the chemical name for Propecia, which I believe works better for women and men in a 5 mg dose, rather than the usually prescribed 1 mg; spironolactone (Aldactone); birth control pills; hormone replacement therapy (estrogen and progesterone); corticosteroids; Flutamide; and Avodart. Avodart is actually a drug used for the treatment of prostate conditions in men; when it was found to have a positive effect on hair loss, it began to be prescribed off-label for use in women.

As with any prescription medications, you must discuss the potential side effects and contraindications with your physician prior to use.

HAIR GROWTH ON THE FACE

Talk about a double whammy. Women of a certain age—well, the age when perimenopause starts—notice to their dismay that their once glorious manes seem to be falling out of their heads even while hair is sprouting on their chin and cheeks. Aren't hormones swell?

Hair growth on the face, which increases with age as hormonal levels shift and decline, can be blamed on those pesky androgens again. (Sudden and/or profuse hair growth on the face should, of course, be examined by a physician.) But many women, especially those of certain ethnicities that tend to be more hirsute, have normal hair growth on their faces, starting with puberty. (Think Frida Kahlo!) The hair might be embarrassing, but it's not a cause for medical concern.

Over-the-Counter (OTC) Skin-Care Products

Many are the products devoted to hair removal: shaving creams, waxes, depilatories, tweezers. They all work temporarily, but they all can cause irritation. (Always test a depilatory for sensitivity on your arm or leg prior to use on your face.) On the other hand, they're extremely inexpensive and easy to use.

I've often corrected that misconception that shaving makes hair grow back thicker or more profusely. It doesn't—but when the hair is growing back, it feels a little stubbly, which is why people think it's coarser.

If you're planning to get waxed, always stop using any prescription retinoids or glycolic acid products in the area where you're going to wax for a week prior to waxing, or you can get a whopping burn.

Prescription Topicals

Vaniqa is a prescription cream that effectively retards hair growth, but it must be used constantly in order to remain effective. A very small percentage of users can get irritated or red. If that happens, discontinue use and consult your dermatologist.

Lasers

Before lasers came along, the only way to permanently remove hair was electrolysis, a painful and tedious procedure where a needle with an electrical current is inserted into each hair follicle to destroy it. Now, thankfully, laser hair removal is big business—which not only gives women more options to deal with unwanted hair, but competition in the market has driven costs way down. The earliest lasers used for hair removal only targeted dark hair on fair skin, but now there are so many different lasers that those with darker skin and hair can be treated. As usual, the effectiveness of the removal and the avoidance of any reactions depends on the skill of the operator and the specific wavelength of the laser. The darker your skin, the longer the wavelength of the laser. A 1064 wavelength laser, like the Lyra, is quite effective on darker skin.

As each hair follicle is independent of the others, hairs are always in different stages of growth and resting. For that reason, multiple treatments are necessary. You'll need to have about six treatments, usually spaced four to six weeks apart, for permanent results.

Lasers cannot work on light hairs, so if you have white or gray hair on your face, you'll have to seek another treatment.

One warning: Do *not* use lasers when you're tan, as the extra melanin interferes with the absorption of the laser's energy into the hair follicle and can cause problems. Use this as yet another good reason to stay out of the sun!

As with all lasers, you can get burned or splotchy. Make sure that whoever's wielding the laser has been well trained in the use of that particular device.

10-Minute Tips

- As there is often a hormonal component to hair loss, be sure to see your doctor to check hormone levels.

- Avoid hairstyles that pull tightly, as that can exacerbate hair loss.

- Use thickening shampoos and conditioners, or shampoos with zinc or anti-fungal agents to reduce inflammation.

- Don't use too many different hair products.

- Find a sympathetic hairstylist who will work with your hair. The better the haircut, the less you'll have to go for trims and touch-ups.

- Test hair-removal products on your arm before using on your face.

- Most of all, don't be too embarrassed to discuss hair loss or hair growth with your dermatologist. There are many treatment options, and you shouldn't suffer in silence!

20

Rosacea and Redness

ROSACEA IS ONE of the most underdiagnosed skin conditions affecting adults. It usually appears after the age of thirty or so. Many, many of my older patients have it, yet are completely unaware that there's a name for their perpetually flushed cheeks. They're shocked when I tell them they have rosacea!

The root cause of rosacea, which affects those with fair to medium skin, especially of Celtic descent, is still unknown. Not surprisingly, this makes finding a permanent cure difficult. Rosacea is a noncontagious vascular condition that appears as redness on the cheeks, nose, chin, or forehead; is often accompanied by small visible blood vessels on the face; and can sometimes be accompanied by acne or watery or irritated eyes. (The pimple component of rosacea erroneously leads people to believe they only have acne, and they can inadvertently use skin-care products that will worsen rosacea. For treatment of adult acne, see chapter 21.) There's often an inflammatory component, leading to a combination of seborrheic dermatitis with rosacea.

Rosacea's symptoms vary considerably. Some of the most common rosacea triggers include sun exposure (you're not surprised about that, are you?), hot or cold weather, wind, alcohol (especially red wine), spicy foods, heavy exercise and sweating, hot baths and saunas, hot drinks, fragrance, hormones, and certain skin-care products. Even when you know your triggers and take care to avoid them, rosacea's flushes can appear with maddening unpredictability. Surveys conducted by the National Rosacea Society found that nearly 70 percent of rosacea sufferers reported that it had lowered their self-confidence and self-esteem, and a staggering 41 percent reported that it had caused them to avoid public contact or cancel social engagements.

Rosacea is usually a progressive disease, which means it needs to be treated—chronically. Once you start treatment, you'll likely be on it for a long time (and sometimes in perpetuity). Fortunately, most patients stick to their protocol. One look at W. C. Fields's bulbous nose, called *rhinophyma*, a thickening of excess tissue as a result of untreated rosacea, is enough to have them renew their prescriptions.

If you find yourself flushed, or if you think you have other symptoms of rosacea, see your dermatologist.

Over-the-Counter (OTC) Skin-Care Products

So many of my rosacea patients were frustrated by the lack of OTC products to help them that I created Laser Relief. The active ingredients include white and green tea, grapeseed extract, and pilewort extract, all of which will help calm skin and reduce redness. You can use it twice a day. Those with oily skin and rosacea can use the Poreless line. See chapter 8 for more information.

If you have rosacea, you need to avoid active, regular exfoliation unless okayed by your dermatologist. That means minimal or no use of home microdermabrasion or peels, as they can increase redness, irritation, and flaking; most of my patients can tolerate them once a month.

Rosacea Creams

B. Kamins Booster Blue Rosacea Treatment

DERMAdoctor Calm Cool & Corrected

Dr. Brandt Laser Relief

Prescription Topicals

Topical anti-inflammatories are prescribed to combat irritation and redness. They include Elidel and Protopic, Noritate, Finacea, Metrogel, sulfur drugs like Klaron, Plexion, or Clenia, or combinations of sulfurs and sodium sulfacetes. (Many people are allergic to sulfur-based drugs, so be aware that there might be reactions.) There may be some side effects, so discuss with your dermatologist.

A new non-steroidal anti-inflammatory cream that has no effect on the immune system, Atopiclair, also shows promising results.

Mechanical Exfoliation

Some patients with rosacea find they can tolerate occasional microdermabrasion, but most can't. No dermabrasion should be performed on anyone with rosacea or a tendency to redness. Irritation will only make you redder!

Intense Pulsed Light, GentleWaves LED, Photodynamic Therapy, Coblation, Thermage, and Titan

IPL is one of the best treatments for rosacea and facial redness, especially if you have fine capillaries and pink matting. Treatment should take only about 20 minutes, and should be done in a series of three to five treatments, two weeks apart.

Once the series is finished, rosacea and redness do tend to gradually return, so be warned that this may be an ongoing treatment. It does have such positive results, though, that you will look much better after treatment. I think it's definitely worth exploring, especially when used in conjunction with topical prescription medications.

Chemical Peels

As with microdermabrasion, peels are forbidden. Any treatment that can cause inflammation may worsen rosacea.

Lasers

Rosacea also responds well to vascular lasers that target blood vessels. Either the Vbeam, Aura, VersaPulse, or Gemini can be used.

10-Minute Regimen

For a woman with rosacea, along with sun damage, loss of resiliency, dry skin, and moderate wrinkles.

A.M.: Preventative

1. Cleanser, eye cream. (Toner is usually not recommended for rosacea, to avoid any irritation.)

2. Rosacea cream: reduces inflammation and calms redness.

3. Anti-oxidant cream: anti-oxidant boost, protects against free-radical damage.

4. Sunscreen.

P.M.: Repair

1. Cleanser, eye cream.

2. Rosacea cream: reduces inflammation and calms redness.

3. Anti-oxidant cream: anti-oxidant boost, protects against free-radical damage.

225

Fredric Brandt, MD

Special Treatments

Home Microdermabrasion: polishes complexion while improving
overall texture of skin. Gently massage on damp skin for two
minutes; rinse. Use every two weeks.

Home Peel: tightens pores, improves firmness, and brightens skin.
Follow instructions in kits. Use every three weeks. Never use on the
same day as home microdermabrasion

ABOUT SENSITIVE SKIN

Many people think they have sensitive skin, when they actually *don't*. Very few
people, only about 2 percent to 3 percent of women, have truly sensitive skin
in the clinical sense. Dermatologists refer to them as "stingers," as their skin
turns red, itches, tingles, and/or burns whenever any products are applied.

The other 97 percent have *inflamed* skin, or seborrheic dermatitis. You
might apply a product and experience stinging and burning due to an underlying inflammation. Perhaps you were overzealous with your microdermabrasion
cream or other exfoliants; perhaps you used a peel that was too strong for your
skin; perhaps you've been spending too much time in the sun. Or you are
using a combination of too many skin-care products, overloading your skin
with a wide range of ingredients that can react with each other. When the inflammation is calmed down, however, the sensitivity disappears.

My patients often complain that they have dry skin that's red and flaky,
and they attribute that to a sensitivity reaction to their skin-care products.
What I tell them is that they need to differentiate between dryness and inflammation. Dry skin will be dry all over your face. It may be a little flaky, but it
won't be red. Inflamed skin usually appears in the central face, around the eyebrows, and it's red. Chronic red skin may well be rosacea, which is not caused
by irritation or skin sensitivity.

Many women also assume they're allergic to certain ingredients if they
have a reaction to a product. They may be right, especially with fragrance, the
most common allergen. Most quality products on the market now, though, are

hypo-allergenic or use natural botanicals with calming properties to mask any rancid or chemical smells.

So, if your skin becomes very red when you apply any products, or simply when you touch it, it's truly sensitive. When this happens, it's a good idea to see a dermatologist to get your skin analyzed, as reactions can persist for weeks, if not months. If you can't do that, look for signs of seborrhea: redness and inflammation around the nose or forehead. Check to see if you have dandruff, because they tend to go hand in hand. Reactions also tend to worsen when you're under stress, so try to keep that to a minimum, too.

10-Minute Tips

- Avoid known triggers whenever possible.

- Bring your skin-care products to the dermatologist so they can be evaluated for possible irritants.

- Don't self-diagnose: Your skin may be irritated, not sensitive, and the products you're using might inadvertently make your skin worse.

- Stick to your prescription regimen, as rosacea may progress without ongoing care. Recognize that it's a chronic condition that needs to be treated.

21

Adult Acne

"OH MY GOD, I'M OLD! I've got wrinkles and acne! How can this be? I thought by the time I got wrinkles, I wouldn't have to live with zits anymore!"

Unfortunately, I hear this lament all too often. But don't blame chocolate, french fries, or the fact that you forgot to wash your face last night. They have nothing to do with acne—in teens or in adults. Blame it on hormones, as the *P. acnes* bacteria that causes acne is primarily due to hormones, as well as genetics. (As women age, one thing they do know a lot about is fluctuating hormones!) Which brings many of them in to see me, unhappy that the skin condition they thought they'd left behind with the end of puberty is once more wreaking havoc on their appearance.

Although the exact cause is still unknown, pimples erupt when the oil (sebaceous) glands become plugged with an excess of oil and dead skin cells. Acne isn't just a condition that happens to teenagers during puberty. Adult acne, like rosacea, is incredibly common. As I discussed in chapter 19, it's sometimes associated with hair loss on the head and hair growth on the face—caused by the declining feminizing hormones and increased masculinizing hormones during perimenopause and menopause. It's not directly caused by stress, but it certainly can be exacerbated by it. Sometimes, too, certain medications or cosmetics can trigger acne, although it should clear right up once the trigger is eliminated.

Like rosacea, acne can progress if not treated. Cystic acne, which produces large cysts and pustules, can leave disfiguring scars. There are many options that you should discuss with your dermatologist, so there's no need to pile on the concealer and suffer in silence.

What works best is often a question of experimentation till the best regimen is found. I often need to combine modalities—prescription topicals, prescription hormones, lasers, and so on—over several months. Obviously, patient compliance is a key factor.

OTC medications can work well on acne, but if it persists, dermatologists should work in tandem with gynecologists; together, we can monitor progress when patients are treated with hormones. There are potential risks and side effects to any hormonal treatment, and these need to be discussed and thoroughly understood. Some medications are toxic to developing fetuses and must be stopped for several months prior to you getting pregnant, and can never be taken during pregnancy.

If acne comes on suddenly, you should always consult your physician or dermatologist, as this may be indicative of an underlying medical condition, such as *polycystic ovarian syndrome.*

Over-the-Counter (OTC) Skin-Care Products

Most of the acne treatments available OTC are formulated for teens, who tend to have very oily skin along with acne. As a result, they may be too harsh and drying for women who tend to have breakouts as well as dry skin.

To treat acne, look for OTC products with flaxseed oil, to decrease oil production, and tea tree oil, which is a natural antibacterial. If you choose quality products, these ingredients should be gentle enough to use every day without drying or irritating your skin. This is especially important, as there's often an inflammatory component to acne as well. Using an OTC anti-irritant product should help reduce redness and irritation.

Home microdermabrasion and peels are also an excellent idea.

Give an OTC regimen at least six to eight weeks to work. If it hasn't made a dent by then, you should consult a dermatologist for prescription treatment.

Fredric Brandt, MD

Prescription Topicals and Medications

The retinoid Differin is a potent treatment. It's the only retinoid that can both reduce inflammation and help unblock pores by removing the dead skin cells that clog them up. Differin may be a little less irritating than Retin-A or Tazorac; start out slowly and see which one has the fewest side effects, such as peeling or drying.

I usually combine a retinoid with a topical antibiotic that often includes benzoyl peroxide and clindamycin. Those with very sensitive skin may use clindamycin on its own, but the advantage of the combination is that it reduces the chance of bacterial resistance.

I've also found that the retinoid Tazorac helps scars. I keep all my acne patients on the Tazorac cream or gel because I truly believe it helps reduce the scars' deepness as well as helping to reduce pore size. You won't see overnight results, but it definitely helps.

If there's an inflammatory and/or rosacea component, I'll prescribe Elidil or Atopiclair. If there's no allergy to sulfur, which is quite common, I may prescribe a sulfur-based drug like Klaron, Plexion, or Clenia, depending on the needs of the patient.

As for hormones, if birth control pills are an option, many women respond well to Yasmin.

If you have severe cystic acne, the much maligned and misunderstood Accutane is still a very good treatment—as long as you are not planning to get pregnant in the near future. Getting the prescription is complicated and regular blood tests are mandatory while you're taking it, but for those who really need it, Accutane can be life-saving, preventing huge scars and deformity.

Sometimes, there are pimples and irritation around the mouth. That may be a form of acne called peri-oral dermatitis, often triggered by the use of certain types of toothpaste, especially whitening and tartar control formulas. A topical anti-inflammatory often helps. This may be combined with oral and/or topical antibiotics.

Dermatologists can also shrink or remove cysts or large pimples with an injection of cortisone or an extraction. Remember this in case you get a huge pimple before an important event!

Mechanical Exfoliation

Microdermabrasion will exfoliate the dead skin cells that clog pores, so it's a good idea to have a series of treatments.

Intense Pulsed Light, GentleWaves LED, Photodynamic Therapy, Coblation, Thermage, and Titan

IPL, amino-levulinic acid (ALA), and blue light treatments help kill the *P. acnes* bacteria and shrink the size of the sebaceous glands.

Injectible Fillers

Fillers can work wonders on distensible acne scars. (You can self-test to see if a scar is distensible: Take your hand and stretch the skin. If the scar goes away, it's distensible.) Silicone is often the filler of choice. Micro-droplets can be injected into the scar, the result is permanent, and the scar will be gone for good. As ever with silicone, make sure your dermatologist has experience with scar treatment.

Ice pick scars or large pores cannot be filled. (Sometimes they can be removed, the scar stitched up, and then either treated with a peel or a laser.)

Chemical Peels

The best types of peels for adult acne contain salicylic acid. As salicylic acid is oil-soluble, it can work directly in pores to clean them, plus it has an anti-inflammatory effect.

I prefer lasers to peels for the treatment of acne scars.

Lasers

Although there is not yet clear data from clinical trials about the ultimate effectiveness of certain lasers for the treatment of adult acne, they may still be a viable option. I've seen good results with the Smoothbeam and Gemini.

Lasers have been proven to have a remarkable affect on acne scars, as their deep heating somehow manages to shrink them. For scarring, I recommend lasers over peels, as they can target specific scars, while peels need to be applied over a larger area. Non-ablative lasers, such as CoolTouch or Smoothbeam, work well. So does Fraxel. Ablative lasers like the Erbium:YAG or CO_2 have also been used, although there is the pain factor and long recuperation time.

10-Minute Regimen

For a woman with oily/combination skin and acne.

A.M.: Preventative

1. Cleanser, toner, eye cream.

2. Pore treatment gel: mattifies shine. Those with mature skin may wish to add an anti-glycation serum before applying pore treatment gel.

3. Skin tightener: tightens and firms skin.

4. Sunscreen.

P.M.: Repair

1. Cleanser, toner, eye cream.

2. Pore treatment cream: clarifying, hydrating treatment that absorbs oil, unclogs pores, and calms redness.

Special Treatments

Mask Treatment: clears blackheads and whiteheads, draws out impurities deep in the skin, balances excess oil secretions, and reduces redness. Use once or twice a week on oily areas. Apply in an opaque layer, avoiding eye area. Leave on for 10 to 15 minutes. Rinse with lukewarm water.

Home Microdermabrasion: polishes complexion while improving overall texture of skin. Gently massage on damp skin for two minutes; rinse. Use once or twice a week, leaving three to four days between treatments.

Home Peel: tightens pores, improves firmness, and brightens skin. Follow instructions in kits. Use every ten days. Never use on the same day as home microdermabrasion.

10-Minute Tips

- Don't pick at pimples—you'll just make them worse.

- Scrubbing skin doesn't help; it just causes more irritation. Don't get too zealous with your cleansing routine!

- Change and wash your pillowcases often, as they can be quickly riddled with unwanted bacteria.

- Stick to the regimen, as it may need to be continued for quite some time, especially if your acne is hormonal. The suggested regimens here will take you less than 10 minutes. And they work!

- Always see a physician if acne comes on suddenly. Hormonal fluctuations do usually respond to some form of treatment. You may, for example, be on a birth control pill that's not the right one for you.

- Chocolate and french fries don't cause acne.

- Sun exposure does not help cure acne—that's a myth.

- Stress doesn't cause acne, but it can exacerbate it.

- Even if you have breakouts, your skin still needs hydration.

APPENDIX 1

Dr. Brandt Cleanse Diet

FOLLOWING A DIET or a cleansing regimen is, of course, naturally beneficial, but it's extremely challenging to devise appropriate recipes that are easy to prepare as well as flavorful. Here are a week's worth that you can mix and match during your cleansing period but are delicious enough for you to want to keep in your recipe repertoire even when your cleansing time is over.

Day 1

Breakfast

8-ounce glass green apple juice

1 cup millet cereal flakes with rice milk and a handful of blueberries

1 slice millet toast

Lunch

Quinoa Salad with Green Beans and Asparagus

2 cups water

1 cup quinoa (pronounced *keen-wah*), rinsed and drained

3 tablespoons lemon juice

Salt and freshly ground pepper to taste

1 pound green beans, trimmed

1 pound asparagus, trimmed

2 tablespoons minced fresh flat-leaf parsley

2 tablespoons minced fresh basil

Mixed baby greens

6 cherry tomatoes, halved

To make the quinoa: In a large saucepan over medium heat, bring water to a boil. Add quinoa, cover, and return to boil. Reduce the heat to simmer, and cook for about 15 minutes or until the quinoa is tender. Transfer to a mixing bowl and toss with the lemon juice. Season with salt and pepper. Let cool to room temperature.

In a large skillet over medium heat, steam the asparagus for 4 to 5 minutes or until tender. Drain and let cool. Cut into ½-inch pieces. In the same skillet, steam the green beans for 4 to 5 minutes or until tender. Drain and let cool. Cut into ½-inch pieces. Toss half the asparagus and half the green beans with half the quinoa. (Cover and refrigerate remaining quinoa, asparagus, and green beans for Day 3, Lunch.) Sprinkle with the parsley and basil. Arrange baby greens on a plate and top with quinoa and vegetables. Surround with cherry tomatoes.

Serves 2

Dinner

Poached Fish with Fresh Salsa

SALSA

8 tomatoes, chopped

1 large onion, chopped

½ cup minced cilantro

¼ cup lime juice

Salt and freshly ground black pepper to taste

FISH

1 cup water

¼ teaspoon salt

10 peppercorns

2 tablespoons chopped onion

2 sprigs fresh flat-leaf parsley

Two 6-ounce white fish fillets (about 1 inch thick)

Mixed baby greens

1 tablespoon lemon juice

To make the salsa: In a medium bowl, combine all the ingredients. Cover and refrigerate for up to 2 days.

Makes 2 cups

To poach the fish: In a large skillet over medium heat, bring the water to a boil. Add the salt, peppercorns, onion, parsley, and fish. Return to boil, then reduce heat to simmer and cook for 7 to 8 minutes, or until the fish flakes easily when tested with a fork. With a spatula, remove the fish from the pan and top each piece with ¼ cup of the salsa. (Cover and refrigerate remaining salsa for Day 2, Lunch.) Serve with mixed baby greens tossed with lemon juice.

Serves 2

Snack

Handful of raw almonds or pistachios

Day 2

Breakfast

8-ounce glass green apple juice

1 slice millet toast

Egg White Omelet with Spinach

Olive oil cooking spray

¼ cup chopped onion

One 5-ounce bag baby spinach, coarsely chopped

1 tablespoon water

4 large egg whites or ¾ cup liquid egg whites

Salt and freshly ground black pepper to taste

Spray a large skillet with olive oil cooking spray. Add the onion and cook over medium heat, stirring frequently, for 2 to 3 minutes or until soft but not browned. Add the spinach and water, and cook, stirring frequently, for 2 to 3 minutes or until the spinach is wilted. Transfer to a colander set over a bowl and drain off excess liquid, gently pressing on the spinach. In a large bowl, whisk together the egg whites, salt, and pepper.

Spray the same skillet with a little more cooking spray. Pour 1 cup of the egg mixture into the skillet and cook, lifting up cooked egg around edge occasionally to let raw egg flow underneath, for about 2 minutes or until the omelet is set but top is still slightly moist. Spoon half of the spinach over half the omelet. Fold remaining half of omelet over filling and cook for 1 to 2 minutes longer. Transfer to a plate and cover with foil to keep warm. Repeat, making one more omelet with remaining egg mixture and spinach.

Serves 2

Lunch

Mixed Bean Salad with Fresh Salsa

1 cup garbanzo beans (see *Note*)

1 cup black beans

1 cup kidney beans

1 cup pinto beans

1 piece kombu

½ cup chopped onion

1 tablespoon minced garlic (optional)

1 tablespoon lemon juice

½ cup Fresh Salsa (see Day 1, Dinner)

Pinch of cumin

Pinch of chili powder

Salt and freshly ground black pepper to taste

Mixed baby greens for serving

If soaking beans overnight: In a large pot, soak the beans in enough water to cover for 12 hours. Drain, rinse, add fresh water, and soak again for 12 hours. Drain, rinse, add fresh water and kombu, and cook over medium heat, partly covered, for 1½ to 2 hours or until tender.

For a quick soak: Place beans in a large pot. Add enough water to cover, bring to a boil with the kombu, and cook for 2 minutes. Remove from heat, cover, and let stand for 1 hour. Drain water and beans.

In a large bowl, combine the cooked beans, onion, garlic (if using), lemon juice, and salsa. Season with cumin, chili powder, salt, and pepper and toss well. Arrange greens on a plate and top with the bean salad.

Serves 2

Note: Dry beans, soaked and cooked as above, are preferable to canned beans. If you wish, you can double the amount, cover, and refrigerate the remaining beans for another recipe.

Dinner

Oven-Poached Salmon with Vegetables and Brown Rice

BROWN RICE

1 cup uncooked brown rice

2¼ cups water

½ teaspoon salt

POACHED FISH

½ cup organic no-salt chicken broth

¼ cup thinly sliced fennel bulb (about 1 small bulb)

3 thyme sprigs

1 garlic clove, minced

⅓ cup water

¼ cup diced celery

¼ cup diced red pepper

Two 6-ounce salmon fillets (about 1 inch thick)

Pinch of salt

Freshly ground black pepper to taste

To make the rice: In a large saucepan over medium heat, combine the rice, water, and salt. Bring to a boil, stir once, and then cover with a tight-fitting lid. Reduce heat to low and cook for about 45 minutes or until rice is tender. Remove from heat and let stand, covered, for 5 to 10 minutes longer.

Makes about 3 cups

Preheat the oven to 325°F. In a large skillet over medium-low heat, combine the chicken broth, fennel, thyme, garlic, and water. Bring to a simmer, cover, and cook for 5 minutes. Stir in the celery and pepper. Cook for 1 minute, then remove from the heat.

Sprinkle the salmon with salt and pepper. Place fillets, skin side up, over vegetable mixture in pan. Cover with a lid and wrap the handle with foil. Bake for 15 minutes, or until the fish flakes easily when tested with a fork. Discard skin and thyme sprigs. Arrange salmon and fennel mixture on individual plates and drizzle with a little of the cooking liquid. Serve with ½ cup brown rice. (Cover and refrigerate remaining brown rice for Day 4, Dinner.)

Serves 2

Snack

1 cup steamed edamame (pronounced *ed-ah-MAH-may*) pods

Day 3

Breakfast

8-ounce glass green apple juice

1 cup millet cereal flakes with rice milk and a handful of blueberries

1 slice millet toast

Lunch

White Bean Soup

> Olive oil cooking spray
>
> 2 tablespoons minced garlic
>
> 2 tablespoons chopped onion
>
> 1 celery stalk, chopped
>
> 2 cups white beans
>
> 1 cup water
>
> Salt and freshly ground black pepper to taste
>
> Pinch dried rosemary
>
> Pinch dried oregano
>
> 1 teaspoon lemon juice
>
> Quinoa Salad for serving (see Day 1, Lunch)

Spray a large saucepan with olive oil cooking spray. Add the garlic, onion, and celery and cook over medium heat, stirring frequently, for 2 to 3 minutes or until soft but not browned. Soak the beans as suggested on page 238 (Day 2, Lunch). Add the beans, water, salt, pepper, rosemary, and oregano. Reduce heat to medium-low and cook for 18 to 20 minutes or until all the vegetables are tender and the soup is hot. Stir in the lemon juice.

Working in batches, transfer the soup to a food processor or blender and purée until smooth. Or use an immersion blender and purée in the pan. Return the soup to the pan to reheat. Serve half with Quinoa Salad. (Cover and refrigerate remaining soup for Day 5, Lunch.)

Serves 2

Dinner

Poached Chicken with Brown Rice Spaghetti, Wilted Kale, and Pine Nuts

CHICKEN

1 cup water

1 cup reduced-sodium chicken broth

½ cup chopped onion

1 stalk celery, chopped

2 garlic cloves, minced

1 bay leaf

10 peppercorns

Four 6-ounce skinless, boneless chicken breast halves

6 ounces (½ package) spaghetti-style brown rice pasta

SPINACH AND PINE NUTS

Olive oil cooking spray

½ bunch kale, trimmed and chopped

1 tablespoon water

½ cup pine nuts

To poach the chicken: In a large skillet over medium heat, combine the water, chicken broth, onion, celery, garlic, bay leaf, and peppercorns. Bring to a boil, then reduce the heat to low and simmer for 15 minutes. Add the chicken to pan, bring to a boil, then reduce heat to low and simmer for 5 minutes. Remove the pan from heat, cover, and let stand 30 minutes.

Cook the pasta according to package directions. Rinse with cold water and drain.

To make the kale: Spray a large skillet with olive oil cooking spray. Add the kale and water and cook, stirring frequently, for 3 to 5 minutes or until the kale is wilted. Stir in the pine nuts.

With a slotted spoon, remove the chicken from the pan. Serve one piece of chicken per person with the pasta and kale. (Cover and refrigerate remaining chicken for Day 4, Lunch.)

Serves 2

Snack

1 cup blueberries

Day 4

Breakfast

8-ounce glass green apple juice

1 slice millet toast

Spicy Scrambled Eggs

> Olive oil cooking spray
>
> ¼ cup chopped onion
>
> ½ cup chopped tomatoes
>
> 1 tablespoon minced, seeded jalapeño chili
>
> ½ cup chopped yellow squash
>
> 4 large eggs
>
> Salt and freshly ground pepper to taste
>
> 2 tablespoons minced fresh cilantro

Spray a large skillet with olive oil cooking spray. Add the onion, chili, and squash and cook over medium heat, stirring frequently, for 2 to 3 minutes or until the vegetables are soft but not browned. In a large bowl, whisk together the eggs, salt, and pepper. Add the eggs to the skillet and with a spatula, stir for 4 to 5 minutes or until almost set. Add the tomatoes and cilantro. Stir again and cook for 2 minutes more or until the eggs are set. Serve immediately.

Serves 2

Lunch

Poached Chicken and Asparagus Salad

> ½ pound asparagus, trimmed
>
> Poached Chicken (see Day 3, Dinner)

1 teaspoon minced fresh tarragon

2 tablespoons lemon juice

Salt and freshly ground pepper to taste

Mixed baby greens

6 cherry tomatoes, halved

In a large skillet over medium heat, steam the asparagus for 4 to 5 minutes or until tender. Drain and let cool. Cut the chicken into ½-inch pieces. In a bowl, toss the asparagus and chicken with the tarragon and lemon juice. Season with salt and pepper. Arrange the baby greens on a plate. Top with the asparagus and chicken and surround with the cherry tomatoes.

Serves 2

Dinner

Chili with Brown Rice

Olive oil cooking spray

2 tablespoons minced garlic

2 tablespoons chopped onion

2 tablespoons chopped red pepper

2 tablespoons chopped green pepper

2 cups pinto beans

2 cups kidney beans

3 cups canned chopped tomatoes with juice

2 tablespoons minced fresh basil

3 tablespoons chili powder

Salt and freshly ground pepper to taste

Brown Rice for serving (see Day 2, Dinner)

Soak the beans as suggested on page 238 (Day 2, Lunch). Spray a large saucepan with olive oil spray. Add the garlic, onion, and pepper and cook over medium heat, stirring frequently, for 2 to 3 minutes or until the vegetables are soft but not browned. Add the beans and tomatoes, cover, and bring to a boil. Reduce the heat to medium-low, stir in the basil, chili, salt, and pepper, and simmer for 15 to 20 minutes. Meanwhile, reheat the brown rice. Serve half the chili with the rice. (Cover and refrigerate remaining chili for Day 7, Lunch.)

Serves 2

Snack

Handful of sunflower seeds

Dr. Brandt Cleanse Diet

Day 5

Breakfast

8-ounce glass green apple juice

1 cup millet cereal flakes with rice milk and a handful of blueberries

1 slice millet toast

Lunch

White Bean Soup with Quinoa

> 2 cups water
>
> Salt to taste
>
> 1 cup quinoa, rinsed and drained
>
> Freshly ground black pepper
>
> White Bean Soup (see Day 3, Lunch)

To make the quinoa: In a medium saucepan over medium heat, bring the water to a boil. Add the salt and quinoa, cover, reduce heat to medium low, and cook for 12 to 15 minutes or until tender. Season with pepper. Reheat the White Bean Soup and serve with the quinoa.

Serves 2

Dinner

Oven-Poached Salmon with Edamame "Fried" Rice

"FRIED" RICE

> Olive oil cooking spray
>
> 2 tablespoons chopped onion

2 tablespoons chopped celery

2 tablespoons chopped red pepper

1½ cups shelled frozen edamame

2 cups cooked brown rice

½ cup soy sauce

POACHED FISH

½ cup reduced-sodium chicken broth

¼ cup thinly sliced fennel bulb (about 1 small bulb)

3 sprigs thyme

1 garlic clove, minced

⅓ cup water

¼ cup diced green pepper

¼ cup diced red pepper

Two 6-ounce salmon fillets (about 1 inch thick)

Pinch of salt

Freshly ground black pepper to taste

To make the rice: Spray a large skillet with olive oil cooking spray. Add the onion, celery, and pepper and cook over medium heat for 3 to 5 minutes or until the vegetables are soft but not browned. Add the edamame and continue to cook for 1 minute. Stir in rice and soy sauce. Keep warm.

To make the salmon: Preheat the oven to 325°F. In a large skillet over medium-low heat, combine the chicken broth, fennel, thyme, garlic, and water. Bring to a simmer, cover, and cook for 5 minutes. Stir in the pepper. Cook for 1 minute, then remove from the heat. Sprinkle the salmon with salt and pepper. Place fillets, skin side up, over vegetable mixture in pan. Cover with a lid and wrap the handle with foil. Bake for 15 minutes or until the fish flakes easily when tested with a fork. Discard skin and thyme sprigs. Serve immediately with the rice.

Serves 2

Snack

Handful of raw almonds or pistachios

Day 6

Breakfast

8-ounce glass green apple juice

1 slice millet toast

Veggie Egg White Omelet

Olive oil cooking spray

2 tablespoons chopped onion

3 large white mushrooms, diced

½ zucchini, chopped

½ red pepper, de-seeded and chopped

4 large egg whites or ¾ cup liquid egg whites

Salt and freshly ground pepper to taste

Avocado slices for serving

Spray a large skillet with olive oil cooking spray. Add the onion, mushrooms, red pepper, and zucchini and cook, stirring frequently, for 2 to 3 minutes or until the vegetables are soft but not browned. In a large bowl, whisk together the egg whites, salt, and pepper.

Spray the same skillet with a little more cooking spray. Pour ½ of the egg mixture into the skillet and cook, lifting up cooked eggs around the edge occasionally to let raw egg flow underneath, for about 2 minutes or until omelet is set but top is still slightly moist. Spoon half of the vegetables over half of omelet. Fold remaining half of omelet over filling and cook for 1 to 2 minutes longer. Transfer to a plate and cover with foil to keep warm. Repeat, making 1 more omelet with remaining egg mixture and vegetables. Surround with avocado slices.

Serves 2

Lunch

Salade Niçoise with Edamame

Olive oil cooking spray

8 ounces fresh tuna

Salt and freshly ground black pepper

½ pound green beans, trimmed

1 cup blanched edamame

Mixed baby greens

½ cup red onion, thinly sliced

6 cherry tomatoes, halved

2 tablespoons lemon juice

2 tablespoons minced fresh flat-leaf parsley

Spray a large skillet with olive oil cooking spray. Sprinkle the tuna with salt and pepper. Cook the tuna over medium heat for 4 minutes on each side, or until the fish flakes easily when tested with a fork. Remove from the pan and let cool.

In a large skillet over medium heat, steam the green beans for 4 to 5 minutes or until tender. Drain and let cool. Cook the edamame according to package directions. Break the fish into large chunks. Arrange the greens on a plate. Top with the tuna, cherry tomatoes, green beans, edamame, and onion. Sprinkle with the lemon juice and parsley and a few additional grinds of pepper.

Serves 2

Dinner

Poached Rosemary Chicken with Slow-Roasted Endive

SLOW-ROASTED ENDIVE

6 endive, halved lengthwise, hearts removed

Olive oil cooking spray

Sea salt and freshly ground black pepper to taste

3 to 4 sprigs fresh thyme

CHICKEN

1 cup water

1 cup reduced-sodium chicken broth

½ cup chopped onion

1 stalk celery, chopped

1 sprig fresh rosemary

2 garlic cloves, minced

10 peppercorns

Two 6-ounce skinless, boneless chicken breast halves

To make the endive: Preheat the oven to 350°F. Place the endive in a shallow pan, cut side up. Spray a little olive oil cooking spray over the endive and season with salt and pepper, Tuck the thyme sprigs in between. Roast for about 30 to 40 minutes or until the endive begins to brown. Brush the endive with the pan juices 2 to 3 times while roasting.

Makes 2 side dish servings

To poach the chicken: In a large skillet over medium heat, combine the water, chicken broth, onion, celery, rosemary, garlic, and peppercorns. Bring to a boil, and then reduce the heat to low and simmer for 15 minutes. Add the chicken to the pan, bring to a boil, and then reduce heat to low and simmer for 5 minutes. Remove the pan from heat, cover, and let stand 30 minutes.

Snack

1 cup blueberries

Day 7

Breakfast

8-ounce glass green apple juice

1 cup millet cereal flakes with rice milk and a handful of blueberries

1 slice millet toast

Lunch

Chili with Mixed Vegetable Salad

1 cup asparagus

1 cup green beans

½ cucumber, peeled, seeded, and chopped

1 cup raw broccoli florets

2 tablespoons chopped red onion

6 radishes, sliced

2 tablespoons lemon juice

Salt and freshly ground black pepper

4 ounces mixed baby greens

Chili (see Day 4, Dinner)

In a large skillet over medium heat, steam the asparagus for 4 to 5 minutes or until tender. Drain and let cool. Cut into ½-inch pieces. In the same skillet, steam the green beans for 4 to 5 minutes or until tender. Drain and let cool. Cut into ½-inch pieces. In a medium bowl, combine the beans, asparagus, cucumber, broccoli, onion, and radishes. Toss with the lemon juice and season with salt and pepper. Arrange the baby greens on a plate and top with the mixed vegetables. Reheat the Chili and serve with the salad.

Serves 2

Dinner

Poached Fish with Sesame-Herbed Brown Rice

BROWN RICE

2 cups water

1 cup brown rice

Pinch salt

1 cup sesame seeds

¼ cup minced fresh herbs such as parsley, dill, and basil

POACHED FISH

1 cup water

¼ teaspoon salt

10 peppercorns

2 tablespoons chopped onion

2 sprigs fresh flat-leaf parsley

Two 6-ounce white fish fillets (about 1 inch thick)

To make the rice: In a large saucepan over medium heat, bring the water to a boil. Stir in the rice and salt. Return to a boil, then reduce heat to low and cook, covered, for about 45 minutes or until the rice is tender.

Meanwhile, preheat the oven to 300° F. Spread the sesame seeds out on a baking sheet and cook for about 15 minutes or until the seeds have a nutty aroma.

Transfer the rice to a bowl and stir in the herbs and sesame seeds. (Serve half the rice with the fish. Cover and refrigerate remaining rice for another meal.)

Makes about 3 cups

To poach the fish: In a large skillet over medium heat, bring the water to a boil. Add the salt, peppercorns, onion, parsley, and fish. Return to a boil, then reduce the heat to simmer and cook for 7 to 8 minutes or until the fish flakes easily when tested with a fork. Serve immediately with the herbed rice.

Serves 2

Snack

Handful of raw almonds or pistachios

Recipes written by Margaret Johnson

Ingredients and How They Affect Your Skin

allantoin: prevents irritation to the skin.

aloe vera: healing emollient that soothes irritations and prevents scarring.

anti-oxidants: will boost the skin's strength to protect against free-radical attack and prevent and repair damage from skin's biggest enemy, the sun. They firm, smooth, and stimulate collagen production.

argireline: stimulates collagen production.

avobenzone: full-spectrum protection against UVA and UVB radiation.

bentonite: the most natural detoxifying agent available. It absorbs toxins and delivers nutrients to the skin.

bilberry extract (*Vaccinium myrtillus* extract): calms skin and promotes healthy blood flow to the skin.

bismuth oxychloride: has an absorbing and smoothing effect.

blue-green algae: a rich source of vitamin E, zinc, iron, and copper, with a soothing effect on skin.

chamomile (*Anthemis nobilis* flower oil): calms, soothes, and reduces irritation associated with blemished skin.

citric acid: helps to dissolve oil and debris and unclog pores.

citroflavonoids: a lightening agent based on citrus extracts (lemon peel); powerful anti-oxidant to protect against free-radical damage.

coenzyme Q10 and vitamin C: combination that firms and reenergizes healthy cellular activity, boosts collagen to regain elasticity, and lightens dark circles.

collagen: a protein that gives structure to skin, bones, and teeth and aids in the absorption of iron.

diacetylboldine: slows down production of melanin after UV exposure, giving the skin a lighter, more even pigmentation.

eugenol: local antiseptic with a cooling effect on the skin.

flavonoids (commonly known as bioflavonoids): powerful anti-oxidants providing remarkable protection against free-radical damage.

flax (linum) seed extract: reduces oil production.

fullerenes: spherical sponges that stop action of UVA and UVB by absorbing free radicals.

gamma amino butyric acid (GABA): causes an immediate and visible smoothing effect on the skin.

geranium: known for its soothing and astringent action on the skin. Also helpful in treating acne, bruises, capillaries, burns, and eczema.

ginger (*Zingiber officinale*): reduces inflammation.

glycerin: a humectant, attracting water.

glyceryl distearate (inflacin): non-steroidal anti-inflammatory combined with cooling agents that reduces burning sensation as well as calms redness.

glycolic acid: stimulates cellular renewal to improve texture of skin, leaving it softer and smoother.

grapefruit extract: energizes and regenerates skin.

grapeseed extract (*Vitis vinifera*): powerful anti-oxidant; when combined with green tea, it increases intracellular levels of vitamin C and slows destruction of collagen caused by environmental damage.

green tea (*Camellia sinensis*): anti-inflammatory and anti-oxidant that boosts sunscreen action to protect against free-radical damage. Aside from anti-inflammatory properties, green tea has been clinically proven to be one of the only natural ingredients that can actually prevent cellular damage caused by exposure to UV rays.

guarana: has an energizing effect on the skin.

gynostemma: anti-oxidant, anti-aging, anti-inflammatory.

Hamamelis virginiana (witch hazel): skin freshener, local anesthetic, and gentle astringent.

homosalate octyl: protects you from the sun by absorbing the ultraviolet (UV) and visible sun rays. Reflects, scatters, and absorbs UV rays.

hyaluronic acid: an essential component of the skin's support tissue. Plumps up the skin by holding water up to a thousand times its weight in natural moisture, making it an excellent hydrating agent.

hydroxyprolisilane C: slows glycation process (excess sugar attacking collagen and elastin fibers, causing cells to stiffen and making skin more vulnerable to wrinkling, sagging, and UV damage), protecting network of collagen and elastin and making them more resilient to free radicals.

kaolin: purest and most versatile soft clay, renowned for its detoxifying effect on the skin; promotes a purifying action.

kola: assists in the absorption and action of other ingredients in the skin.

lactic acid: derived from sour milk. Has intense hydrating properties.

lavender: soothing and calming to even out skin's redness and discoloration.

licorice: known for its anti-inflammatory and anti-bacterial properties.

lohan: patented extract from the fruit (member of the squash family) that is intensely sweet and helps reduce cravings for sugar. Known as the longevity fruit.

marine extract: hydrating complex that provides soothing benefits.

matrix metallo proteinases (MMP): an enzyme responsible for the breakdown of collagen.

methyl methacrylate: microspheres that diffuse light, making the appearance of the skin smoother and more uniform.

octyl methoxycinnamate (octinoxate): organic UVB absorber that offers broad protection.

oxybenzone: waterproof UVA/ UVB absorber that is quite stable and enhances the effectiveness of other UVB absorbers.

papaya: balances the skin as well as smoothes irregularities.

phospholipids: binds water and has a long-lasting effect on skin's moisture.

pilewort extract (*Ranunculus ficaria*): anti-inflammatory.

Pisum sativum (sweet pea): a protein derived from the sweet pea plant that produces a tensing, toning, and firming effect on the skin.

polyphenols: increase the strength of the blood vessels by boosting micro-circulation, protecting elastin and collagen fibers, and preventing the destruction of hyaluronic acid, an essential component of the skin's support tissue.

pro-dimethylsilanediol salicylate (salicylic acid family): soothing anti-inflammatory ingredient that restores pH balance in the skin, absorbs oil, and prevents future breakouts.

rice bran oil: has impressive ability to impart a healthy glow to the skin.

rosemary (*Rosmarinus officinalis*): acts as a tonic, or astringent, which is effective for treating combination and oily skins.

saccharide isomerate (Pentavitin): a sugar derivative that binds moisture.

salicylic acid: lipid-soluble beta-hydroxy acid, a non-irritating ingredient that controls excess oil to treat acne while unclogging pores.

salix alba (willow bark): calms irritated skin.

shea butter (*Butyrospermum parkii*): obtained from shea nuts. Moisturizer that has powerful anti-oxidant action.

silicone: allows for rapid absorption and an impressive ultra-lightweight, quick dry-down.

soy protein: resurfaces skin to make it smoother and reduces collagen degradation.

squalane: moisturizer similar to lipids in the skin.

sunflower (*Helianthus annuus*): yields an oil with moisturizing and protective properties.

tea tree oil: an anti-bacterial, lipid-soluble, non-irritating, clarifying ingredient used to treat acne-prone skin.

TIMP-2 (oligopeptide-20): tissue inhibitor of MMP-2. Protects and prevents the depletion of collagen while preserving moisture and elasticity in the skin, delaying the aging process, and prolonging cell life.

titanium dioxide: an active "physical" block micronized and encapsulated in a silicone molecule, ensuring a lightweight, smooth application that leaves none of the usual white traces.

tyrosinase: key enzyme of melanin synthesis.

urea: ingredient that attracts water and holds it in the skin for better hydration.

vitamin A (retinyl palmitate): increases cell turnover, helps to stimulate collagen production, keeps pores from clogging, and lightens discoloration on the skin.

vitamin C, vitamin E: powerful anti-oxidants that protect cells against free-radical damage due to sun exposure. An added protection against UVA (aging) and UVB (burning) rays. Also provide hydration while restoring firmness and elasticity.

vitamins A and C: together, they encourage cell renewal.

white tea (*Camellia sinensis*): potent anti-oxidant that protects skin against free-radical damage.

willow bark (*Salix alba*): calming and cooling agent.

zinc: an active physical filter that blocks sun's rays, extracted from the chamomile plant. Helps calm inflammation and redness.

zinc oxide: helps calm redness and irritation.

INDEX

Index

ABOUT THE AUTHOR

FOR MORE THAN TWENTY YEARS, Dr. Fredric Brandt has been revolutionizing the field of cosmetic dermatology. He was the first to introduce green tea into skin care and the first to launch at-home treatments—such as Dr. Brandt Microdermabrasion, Dr. Brandt Laser Tight, and Dr. Brandt Laser A-Peel—that mimic in-office procedures. This internationally known lecturer, innovative researcher, and sought-after physician is revered by patients, prestigious medical companies, and colleagues alike.

Dr. Brandt is the foremost leader when it comes to injectibles, currently recognized as the biggest user of the most innovative age-fighters, such as Restylane and Botox. He revolutionized the industry when he moved beyond the traditional uses of Botox to create the Botox neck lift and the Botox nose lift. This cutting-edge, artistic approach to utilizing cosmetic dermatological treatments, combined with his extensive knowledge of cosmetic dermatology and his groundbreaking in-office procedures, has made Dr. Brandt famous within the skin-care industry and beyond it.

A celebrity in his own right, Dr. Brandt has earned the trust of boldfaced names in the worlds of entertainment, business, fashion, and society. Not only do his patients rely on him to keep them looking close-up–ready, but they also admire him as an artist, as he helps them sculpt the younger appearance they seek. Using a variety of noninvasive procedures, many of which he pioneered or perfected, he helps them maintain their youthful visages.

When he is not seeing patients in his Miami or New York City practice, Dr. Brandt is providing insight and expertise in dermatological research as well as treatment and diagnosis. He currently sits on the advisory board of Artes Medical, and he is a consultant and investigator for such prestigious medical companies as Medicis Aesthetics, Dermik, ColBar LifeScience, Contura, and

Allergan. He is also one of the first dermatologists enlisted by the makers of such revolutionary materials as Restylane, Perlane, Aquamid, Isolagen, Reloxin, CosmoDerm, and CosmoPlast to conduct FDA-approved clinical trials at his Dermatology Research Institute. Beyond this contribution to the field, Dr. Brandt has published numerous professional papers, conducted in-depth industry-wide research programs, is a board-certified member of the American Board of Internal Medicine and the American Board of Dermatology, and holds memberships in prestigious professional societies at both the regional and national levels.

Dr. Brandt's love of skin care started at Memorial Sloan-Kettering Hospital, where as a student he specialized in the research and treatment of leukemia. There he dedicated his studies to using natural ingredients to fight against the growth of cancer. Green tea, vitamin A, and vitamin C became studied treatments under Dr. Brandt's expert eye, and would become the basis of his eponymous skin-care line.

In addition to professional papers, Dr. Brandt is the author of *Age-Less: The Definitive Guide to Botox, Collagen, Lasers, Peels, and Other Solutions for Flawless Skin* (William Morrow, 2002), a revolutionary skin-care manual that contains advice and information from the master of youth himself on how to achieve perfect, youthful skin at any age.

Dr. Brandt regularly appears on *Live with Regis & Kelly*, *Today*, and various other entertainment programs, and both he and his products are regularly featured in top national magazines and newspapers.